O A P L
OXFORD AMERICAN PALLIATIVE CARE LIBRARY

Palliative Aspects of Emergency Care

O A P L
OXFORD AMERICAN PALLIATIVE CARE LIBRARY

Palliative Aspects of Emergency Care

Edited by

Paul L. DeSandre, DO
U.S. Department of Veterans Affairs Medical Center
Assistant Professor, Department of Emergency Medicine

Assistant Chief, Section of Palliative Care—Atlanta VAMC
Emory University School of Medicine Atlanta, Georgia

Tammie E. Quest, MD
U.S. Department of Veterans Affairs Medical Center
Roxann Arnold Professor in Palliative Medicine
Director, Emory Palliative Care Center
Associate Professor, Emergency Medicine
Chief, Section of Palliative Care—Atlanta VAMC
Emory University School of Medicine
Atlanta, Georgia

Executive Series Editor

Russell K. Portenoy, MD
Chairman of the Department of Pain Medicine & Palliative Care
Beth Israel Medical Center
New York, NY

OXFORD
UNIVERSITY PRESS

OXFORD

UNIVERSITY PRESS

Oxford University Press is a department of the University of Oxford.
It furthers the University's objective of excellence in research, scholarship,
and education by publishing worldwide.

Oxford   New York
Auckland   Cape Town   Dar es Salaam   Hong Kong   Karachi
Kuala Lumpur   Madrid   Melbourne   Mexico City   Nairobi
New Delhi   Shanghai   Taipei   Toronto

With offices in
Argentina   Austria   Brazil   Chile   Czech Republic   France   Greece
Guatemala   Hungary   Italy   Japan   Poland   Portugal   Singapore
South Korea   Switzerland   Thailand   Turkey   Ukraine   Vietnam

Oxford is a registered trademark of Oxford University Press in the UK
and certain other countries.

Published in the United States of America by
Oxford University Press
198 Madison Avenue, New York, NY 10016

Library of Congress Cataloging-in-Publication Data
Palliative aspects in emergency care / edited by Paul L. DeSandre and Tammie E. Quest.
    p. ; cm.—(Oxford American palliative care library)
Includes bibliographical references and index.
ISBN: 978–0–19–989561–8 (alk. paper)
I. DeSandre, Paul L.   II. Quest, Tammie E.   III. Series: Oxford American palliative care
library.
[DNLM: 1. Palliative Care.   2. Emergency Service, Hospital.   3. Evidence-Based
Medicine.   4. Hospice Care. WB 310]
616.029—dc23   2012041603

9 8 7 6 5 4 3 2 1
Printed in the United States of America
on acid-free paper

We would like to dedicate this book to the pioneers of emergency care and the patients and families that have informed the work.

Contents

Foreword

"Don't just do something. Stand there."

In 1994, this was my instruction to an emergency medicine trainee prepared to intubate an emaciated, elderly female with fever and dyspnea who was transferred from a nursing home to Grady Memorial Hospital. The rattling cough, evidence of aspiration pneumonia, in a patient with a gastrostomy tube and history of recurrent aspiration, was evidence of the expected inevitable and irreversible course for this woman with a chronic, life-limiting condition.

In this case, it was Alzheimer's dementia, but it might as easily have been cancer, end-stage heart failure, or chronic obstructive pulmonary disease. A call to the family allowed us to hear the patient's wishes as echoed through those who shared her life and her intentions. Our subsequent care honored her wishes and eased her symptoms as she was allowed a natural death, rather than providing her our "heroic" standard of care at the time, one that routinely involved intubation, intensive care unit admission, vasopressors, multisystem organ failure, iatrogenic delirium, and death.

Over the past two decades, I have studied the treatment of pain and other symptoms in our emergency departments and, increasingly, my work has focused on attempts to change the practice of emergency-department-based palliative care. Along the way, I've been privileged to meet exceptional colleagues, and now fast friends, who share these interests, including Drs. Paul DeSandre and Tammie Quest. Thus, it was with great pride that I accepted their kind invitation to provide the foreword for *Palliative Aspects in Emergency Care*, the first text devoted to the emerging subdiscipline of palliative medicine within emergency medicine. *Palliative Aspects in Emergency Care* is a landmark publication that belongs on the shelf of emergency care providers who seek to provide higher quality palliative care to our patients. In other words, all of us should purchase this book and promote it to our colleagues.

In the 1990s, as Medical Director of Grady Memorial Hospital in Atlanta and Associate Chief of what was then the Division of Emergency Medicine at Emory University, we began recruiting a new generation of physicians to rebuild Emory's emergency medicine program and move it toward departmental status. We were fortunate to attract a highly talented group of applicants, including Dr. Tammie Quest. After completing her residency at Highland General Hospital in Oakland, Tammie joined the Emory faculty and received increasing recognition for her mastery of delivering "bad news." Over the past 20 years, Dr. Quest has trained a generation of emergency physicians to do well what had been a haphazard art, at best.

In 2006, Tammie spearheaded our successful effort to lobby the American Board of Emergency Medicine to cosponsor the new specialty of Hospice and Palliative Medicine, thereby including emergency medicine training as a recognized pathway to board certification in palliative medicine. Since that time, a new cadre of emergency physicians, with additional specialty training in palliative medicine, has become board-certified in both specialties. Many of these dual-boarded specialists have joined our academic training programs and have become a driving force to establish higher levels of quality in both generalist and specialty-level palliative care in our departments.

After moving to New York to join the faculty at the Albert Einstein College of Medicine, I established the Pain and Emergency Medicine Institute at Beth Israel Medical Center in Manhattan. There I met Paul DeSandre, a mid-career emergency physician who had developed a passion for palliative care and sought more meaning in his professional life. Paul was accepted into the palliative care fellowship program at Beth Israel and, while remaining an emergency medicine faculty member, completed a two-year, half-time fellowship under the direction of Russ Portenoy, my research mentor and Chair of the first Department of Pain Medicine and Palliative Care in the country. On passing the new Hospice and Palliative Medicine board exam, Dr. DeSandre became one of the first dual-board-certified physicians trained in both an emergency medicine residency and palliative medicine fellowship. He subsequently joined my former colleagues at Emory, where Dr. Quest has established a truly innovative emergency medicine palliative care program.

The emergency department is a crucial setting for identifying unmet palliative care needs and initiating end-of-life discussions with patients, families, and primary care physicians. Think about the number of patients you have seen within the past month whose palliative care needs are not being met. How recently have you treated a patient with a chronic, life-limiting illness who is caught in a revolving door of emergency care, cycling from one acute episode to the next—from the ED to a hospital bed and back to home or a long-term care facility, without being offered palliative care services that could better ease distressing symptoms, improve coordination of services, and provide caregiver relief? Critical actions we take in the emergency department can recognize patient's wishes, and determine subsequent goals and trajectories of care, including appropriate levels of hospital care (including intensive care utilization), and the need for specialty-level palliative care services and hospice.

Palliative Aspects in Emergency Care provides you with a toolkit to meet the needs of your patients with life-limiting illness and injury. Key elements of patient and family assessment; communications with patients, family members, loved ones, and consulting services; care for specific emergent conditions and symptoms, including pain; and, structural and legal issues surrounding palliative care are detailed in a user-friendly format. Additional support for those planning ED-based palliative care quality-improvement initiatives can be accessed through the Improving Palliative Care in Emergency Medicine (IPAL-EM) Project. In 2011, a number of experts in emergency medicine, palliative care, emergency nursing, and social work were brought together by the Center to Advance Palliative Care to develop a catalogue of helpful items, including background documents on the need for ED-based palliative care, sample presentations to help make the case to hospital leadership, needs assessment instruments, lists of key operational, clinical and satisfaction metrics, as well as palliative care screening instruments. The site even includes a plan for accomplishing four things in one week to jump-start the process. These IPAL-EM resources can be accessed through the project Web site (http://www.capc.org/ipal).

In contrast to the clinical inertia implied by my instruction to a resident in the 1990s, I now implore you, my colleagues in emergency care: Don't just stand there. Do something! First, buy this book and read it. Buy copies for all members of your practice group or trainees in your residency program. Buy copies for all emergency nurses in your department. Study its contents in small groups and identify champions for palliative care from hospital administrative and clinical leadership. Open channels of communication with your hospital's palliative care service, local hospice, and clergy. *Palliative Aspects in Emergency Care* arms you with the knowledge to become the problem-solvers emergency physicians pride themselves to be.

A variety of forces bode well for enhanced provision of palliative care by emergency physicians, including changes in population demographics, unsustainable healthcare expenditures, and the development of physicians with dual-specialization in emergency medicine and palliative medicine. Our specialty can add a strategically important voice to the growing chorus calling for improvements in end-of-life care. *Palliative Aspects in Emergency Care* promotes acquisition of the knowledge and skills that will enable us to meet the needs of our patients with life-limiting illness and injury.

Now, don't just stand there. Do something! Join your colleagues in developing palliative care-aware emergency departments that exemplify the best of our specialty and, most importantly, provide the superior quality of care our patients deserve and expect.

Knox H. Todd, MD, MPH, FACEP
Professor and Chair
Department of Emergency Medicine
The University of Texas MD Anderson Cancer Center

Preface

With advances in the treatment of acute illnesses and our aging population, crises related to serious illnesses will drive patients in greater numbers into the unfamiliar and often frightening environment of our emergency departments (ED). The necessary approach in Emergency Medicine is to identify and treat life-threatening problems first, and then move on to secondary concerns in order of priority. When patients with life-threatening illnesses present in crisis to the ED, clinicians must simultaneously address physiologic and symptom concerns while rapidly addressing goals of medical intervention. Even with limited information and guidance, all of this must take into consideration the perspectives of the patient and family. It is certainly understandable that clinicians remain challenged in addressing these complex situations skillfully.[1,2]

In the ED, pain and suffering is routinely experienced, life-limiting illnesses are discovered, patients die, and families grieve. Skillful approaches to pain and symptom management in complex illness remain poorly understood. Although excellent communication skills are well-recognized as essential to good practice in Emergency Medicine, discomfort remains in communications related to life-threatening illness. While outcomes remain extremely poor for out-of-hospital cardiac arrests, family presence during cardiopulmonary resuscitation is not routinely practiced, and approaches to disclosing death to these shocked families are inconsistent. Although emergency clinicians may recognize that a patient is unlikely to survive the next hours or days of hospitalization, it remains challenging to confront that awareness and to communicate those concerns to the family of the dying patient. This reluctance can lead to unwanted or unintended interventions that establish a trajectory of prolonging the dying process, usually in an intensive care unit.

Recognizing the need to advance the study and practice of palliative care in our emergency departments, Emergency Medicine emerged as one of the original sponsoring boards to support the new American College of Graduate Medical Education subspecialty of Hospice and Palliative Medicine.[3] This additional training opportunity for Emergency Medicine specialists has fostered further interest and support for structured and rapid approaches to assessments, communications, and interventions needed for excellent care of this increasingly large portion of our patient population.

In 2008, the original curriculum incorporating palliative care principles into routine emergency care was introduced by the Education in Palliative and End of Life Care—Emergency Medicine (EPEC-EM) project.[5] Many of the authors in this book are faculty or have participated in this exceptional program and have utilized several of the principles from EPEC-EM to provide substance and structure to the topics covered in *Palliative Aspects of Emergency Care*.

From prehospital assessment through discharge planning, there is tremendous opportunity to develop new standards and guidelines to improve care for these most vulnerable patients in our emergency departments. In 2011, the Center to Advance Palliative Care launched a highly accessible resource for the practicing clinician to promote these efforts with the Improving Palliative Care in Emergency Medicine (IPAL-EM) project.[4]

Palliative Aspects of Emergency Care was developed to help the practicing clinician in real time to address real situations skillfully and efficiently. *Palliative Aspects of Emergency Care* uses a practical framework for multidisciplinary teams to address the most common and most pressing ED clinical situations facing patients and families with palliative care needs.

From students through teaching faculty, and including the full range of inter-disciplinary professionals working within the ED, *Palliative Aspects of Emergency Care* offers a format to assure confident communications and interventions to support optimal care in the ED for patients with severe life-threatening or life-limiting illness. Consulting clinicians and administrative professionals would also benefit from *Palliative Aspects of Emergency Care* by gaining additional perspectives on how best to interface and partner with the ED to improve care for patients and families facing severe life-threatening illness in this difficult environment.

References

1. Smith AK, Fisher J, Schonberg MA, et al. Am I doing the right thing? Provider perspectives on improving palliative care in the emergency department. *Ann Emerg Med.* 2009;54:86–93, 93.e1.

2. Grudzen CR, Richardson LD, Hopper SS, Ortiz JM, Whang C, Morrison RS. Does palliative care have a future in the emergency department? Discussions with attending emergency physicians. *J Pain Symptom Manage.* 2012;43:1–9.

3. Quest TE, Marco CA, Derse AR. Hospice and palliative medicine: new subspecialty, new opportunities. *Ann Emerg Med.* 2009;54:94–102.

4. Center for the Advancement of Palliative Care. Improving Palliative Care in Emergency Medicine. http://www.capc.org/ipal/ipal-em. Accessed October 1, 2012.

5. Emanuel LL, Quest TE, eds. *The Education in Palliative and End-of-life Care of Emergency Medicine (EPEC-EM) Project.* Chicago, IL: EPEC Project, Buehler Center on Aging, Health & Society, Northwestern University; 2008.

Acknowledgments

Paul DeSandre wishes to acknowledge my partner, Michael Ross, for his love and support, Tammie Quest for her vision and inspiration, Knox Todd for his dedication and guidance, and Russell Portenoy, for recognizing and supporting the essential role of Emergency Medicine in Palliative Care.

Contributors

Jean Abbott, MD, MH
Attending Physician, Anschutz
 Medical Center
and
Professor Emerita, Emergency
 Medicine &
Faculty, Center for Bioethics and
 Humanities
University of Colorado School of
 Medicine
Aurora, Colorado

Eric Bryant, MD, FACEP
Medical Director
The Denver Hospice/Optio Health
 Services
Denver, Colorado

**Garrett Chan, PhD, APRN,
FAEN, FPCN, FAAN**
Associate Adjunct Professor
 Department of Physiological Nursing
University of California, San Francisco
and
Lead Advanced Practice Nurse
 & Associate Clinical Director
 Clinical Decision Unit
Stanford Hospital & Clinics
Stanford, California

**Arthur R. Derse, MD, JD,
FACEP**
Director, Center for Bioethics and
 Medical Humanities
Julia and David Uihlein Professor of
 Medical Humanities
Professor of Bioethics and
 Emergency Medicine
Institute for Health and Society
Medical College of Wisconsin
Milwaukee, Wisconsin

Paul L. DeSandre, DO
U.S. Department of Veterans Affairs
 Medical Center
Assistant Professor, Emergency
 Medicine
Assistant Chief, Section of Palliative
 Care—Atlanta VAMC
Emory Palliative Care Center
Emory University
Atlanta, Georgia

Kirsten G. Engel, MD
Research Assistant Professor
Department of Emergency
 Medicine
Northwestern University
Chicago, Illinois

Sangeeta Lamba, MD
Associate Professor of Emergency
 Medicine and Surgery
Director of Medical Education
Director of Palliative Care
Department of Emergency
 Medicine
University of Medicine and Dentistry
 of New Jersey, New Jersey
 Medical School
Newark, New Jersey

Ryan Paterson, MD
Associate Professor, Emergency
 Medicine
University of Colorado, Denver—
 Health Science Center,
Denver Health and Hospital
Denver, Colorado

Jan M. Shoenberger, MD
Associate Professor of Clinical
    Emergency Medicine
Keck School of Medicine of the
    University of Southern California
Residency Director, Emergency
    Medicine
Los Angeles County + USC Medical
    Center
Los Angeles, California

Susan C. Stone, MD, MPH
Clinical Associate Professor of
    Medicine
David Geffen School of Medicine,
    UCLA
Director of Home Visits and
    Outpatient Palliative Care, Region 2
Health Care Partners
Los Angeles, California

Jessica Stetz, MD, MS
Department of Emergency Medicine
Assistant Professor of Emergency
    Medicine
SUNY Downstate Medical Center /
    Kings County Hospital Center
Brooklyn, New York

Audrey Tan, DO
Chief Resident, Department of
    Emergency Medicine
SUNY Downstate Medical Center /
    Kings County Hospital Center
Brooklyn, New York

Lynne M. Yancey, MD
Associate Professor, Department of
    Emergency Medicine
University of Colorado School of
    Medicine
Denver Health Residency in
    Emergency Medicine
Denver, Colorado

Chapter 1

Trajectories and Prognostication in Emergency Care

Garrett Chan, PhD, APRN, FAEN, FPCN, FAAN

Introduction

The emergency department (ED) is a fast-paced and high-stress environment where suboptimal information is obtained quickly.[1] Incorporating palliative care into emergency care is vital because it helps provide holistic care and offers treatments that match patients' wishes for their care. Emergency clinicians are procedure-oriented and often rely on algorithms to determine plans of care due to the fast-paced and crisis environment of the ED. However, considering concepts of palliative care at the same time as treating the distress of a patient can help shape the plan of care and perhaps set the course of hospitalization down different pathways, especially in advanced illness. For example, if a patient with advanced chronic obstructive pulmonary disease (COPD) presents to the ED with a chief complaint of shortness of breath, the airway and breathing are of primary concern. Intubation, bronchodilators, and steroids immediately are part of the respiratory failure algorithm. If the patient wishes to avoid intubation, and has expressed this in an advance directive, then intubation should not be considered and treatment to relieve the dyspnea should be primary in the plan of care. Other reported barriers to implementing palliative care principles in the ED include lack of knowledge of palliative care; lack of resources; lack of communication between the ED and primary care providers; conflict among professionals, patients, and families; attention to the needs of the living patients left little time for bereavement; the ED culture's emphasis on using highly technological care and therapies to stabilize patients versus an emphasis on caring behaviors; and a variety of medicolegal concerns.[2–6]

Early recognition of opportunities for palliative interventions will improve the overall quality of emergency care provided to patients and families. Understanding disease and end-of-life trajectories help clinicians recognize where a patient's clinical condition sits on a continuum and match goals of care with interventions that are helpful in relieving suffering as well as possibly reversing pathology. Therefore, the purpose of this chapter is to review the trajectories of advanced disease and to review prognostic tools that can help

ED clinicians in creating tailored plans of care to match the patient's goals or wishes for care.

Emergency Department and Functional Trajectories

ED Trajectories

Sudden acute illnesses or injuries, or an acute exacerbation of chronic illness, often leave little time for advanced care planning and death preparation.[1] Emergency department clinicians must make rapid decisions in a high-stress and fast-paced environment, often with suboptimal levels of information regarding medical history, care preferences, and goals of care.[1,10–13] In addition, relationships are quickly created among the patient, family, and healthcare providers in a time of crisis.[14–16] The same factors that create the necessity for emergency physicians and nurses to initiate diagnostic and treatment algorithms also may create plans of care that are inappropriate for patients' conditions or that are not consistent with their goals of care. Therefore, research has been conducted to illustrate the common presentations and trajectories of approaching death.[17,18] The ED trajectories of approaching death help emergency clinicians recognize the clinical patterns of how patients die in the ED. With this improved understanding that patients are near the end of their lives, appropriate interventions that may not be resuscitative in nature can be implemented.

Seven trajectories of approaching death in the ED have been identified: (1) dead on arrival; (2) prehospital resuscitation with subsequent ED death; (3) prehospital resuscitation with survival until admission; (4) terminally ill and arrives at the ED; (5) frail and hovering near death; (6) alive and interactive on arrival, but arrests in the ED; (7) potentially preventable death by omission or commission.[18] Table 1.1 describes the key characteristics that can alert emergency clinicians that death is approaching. Table 1.2 reviews the key characteristics of each of the seven trajectories with recommended palliative care interventions appropriate for each trajectory.

Functional Trajectories

The use of dying trajectories helps better conceptualize the care of the dying by putting the patient and his therapeutic response into perspective. Two categories of trajectories are reviewed in this chapter: (1) functional trajectories of approaching death; and (2) the ED trajectories of approaching death. Introduced by Glazier and Strauss in their study of dying hospitalized patients in 1968,[7] the Institute of Medicine[8] with further elaboration and validation by Lunney, Lynn, and Hogan[9] describes four functional trajectories of approaching death. These four trajectories (Figure 1.1) are helpful in understanding the patterns of approaching death from a functional status perspective. The first trajectory is **sudden death**. This occurs when a person who was fully functioning in the community without prior history of any serious disease dies. These persons were generally healthy but then suddenly were stricken by acute illness or injury, such as a catastrophic acute myocardial infarction, motor vehicle crash, or aortic dissection. The **disseminated cancer trajectory** describes

Table 1.1 Signs of Mortality and Factors that Contribute to the Perception of Approaching Death[18]

Mechanism of injury	• Penetrating trauma/gunshot wound to the head • Auto vs. pedestrian at high speed • Stab wound to the heart or multiple stab wounds
Chief xomplaint	• Chest pain • Dyspnea • Abdominal pain • Altered level of consciousness
Physiological indicators and diagnostics findings	• Vital signs (temperature, blood pressure, pulse, respiratory rate, SaO2) • Cardiac rhythm (e.g., ventricular fibrillation, asystole) • Massive intracranial hemorrhage on head CT with midline shift and uncal herniation
Physical examination findings	• Cranial vault disruption • Brain parenchyma outside the cranial vault • Evidence of disseminated intravascular coagulation (DIC) • Lab/radiographic findings suggestive of severe or advanced stage of pathology (e.g., urosepsis, aspiration pneumonia, high-grade subdural hematoma) • Abnormal neurological findings (e.g., pupils fixed and dilated)
Demographic factors	• Developmental indicators (e.g., age, height disproportionate to expected weight)
Patient's sense of impending doom or approaching death	• Patient stating they are "going to die," or "don't let me die." • Clinicians listen to patients when the patient perceives that he/she is going to die (in the absence of a psychiatric problem).
Required procedures	• Cardiopulmonary resuscitation: chest compression, intubation, cardiac pacing. • Rapid, massive transfusions • Subdural hematoma evacuation

the course of a patient who struggles with cancer, maintains function fairly well until the last 2–4 months when he or she then rapidly declines, becomes bed-bound, and then dies due to tumor growth. The **organ failure trajectory** resembles a sine wave: people live with relatively good function with heart failure, COPD, or cirrhosis of the liver; have terrible function during an exacerbation; and if they survive, return to a functional level usually below baseline; but again function relatively well until the next crisis. **Frailty** describes the patient with a slowly progressing fatal disease, such as Alzheimer's dementia or amyotrophic lateral sclerosis. These patients progressively lose function, and then die over a period of many years.

When discussing prognosis in the setting of acute exacerbation of a chronic illness, one can safely say that patients will never be better than their adequately

Table 1.2 Observed ED Death Trajectories, Trajectory Characteristics, and Examples of Palliative Care Interventions[18]

Trajectory	Characteristics	Palliative Care Interventions for the Patient or Family[5,6,10,25,36–38]
1. Dead on arrival	• Patient has injuries/medical conditions incompatible with life. • EMTs provided resuscitative efforts in the field. • Consensus among ED clinicians regarding the finality of death. • Patient declared dead within minutes of arrival to the ED.	Physical/Symptoms • No intervention Psychological & Social • Family witnessed resuscitation • Skillful death notification Spiritual • Chaplain, social worker, or any clinician • Cultural considerations for post-mortem care
2. Pre-hospital resuscitation with subsequent ED death	• Physical examination findings and physiological indicators help to determine that the patient is likely to die. • ED clinicians use all available resources at their disposal in an effort to resuscitate the patient. • Clinicians have concerns about neurological outcome if the patient is resuscitated. • Clinicians and/or family members may have differing opinions that death is imminent. • ED clinicians may, however, continue resuscitation efforts despite obvious signs of death due to other factors (e.g., SIDS, pediatric trauma).	Physical/Symptoms • Consider withholding/withdrawing life-sustaining therapies and medicate for distressing symptoms Psychological & Social • Clarify goals of care and match interventions to the goals of care • Assess for advance directives • Family witnessed resuscitation • Skillful delivery of serious news and/or death notification Spiritual • Chaplain, social worker, or any clinician • Cultural considerations for post-mortem care
3. Pre-hospital resuscitation with survival until admission	• EMTs and ED clinicians use various signs of mortality to achieve perceptions of approaching death.	

3a) Resuscitative efforts are likely to be effective	• ED clinicians strive to save a life due to their perception that the patient is likely to survive. • ED clinicians employ aggressive/invasive/heroic efforts in attempt to resuscitate the patient. • Clinicians do not perceive that death is a probability because they fully engage in resuscitative interventions.	**Symptoms** • Consider pain and symptom medications that will not interfere with hemodynamics (e.g., fentanyl) **Psychological & Social** • Clarify goals of care and match interventions to the goals of care • Assess for advance directives • Determine how decisions are made within the family (patient autonomy vs. shared decision-making) • Family witnessed resuscitation • Skillful delivery of serious news **Spiritual** • Chaplain, social worker, or any clinician

3b) Resuscitative efforts are unlikely to be effective	• Uncertainty as to the ending of a patient's life
	• Resuscitation interventions may have a temporary effect to maintain signs of life.
	• Clinical actions:
	  • Are designed to prove to the family and sometimes to themselves that death is the only possible outcome
	  • Are in agreement with patient's previously stated wishes in an advance directive
	  • Are congruent patient/family wishes or expectations in order to protect the clinician and hospital from litigation
	  • Are congruent with the clinicians' own moral values
	  • Are congruent with acceptable standards of practice in order to protect the clinicians' and hospital's reputation and to avoid litigation
		Symptoms
		• Consider pain and symptom medications that will not interfere with hemodynamics (e.g., fentanyl)
		• Consider withholding/withdrawing life-sustaining therapies and medicate for distressing symptoms
		Psychological & Social
		• Clarify goals of care and match interventions to the goals of care
		• Assess for advance directives
		• Determine how decisions are made within the family (patient autonomy vs. shared decision-making)
		• Family witnessed resuscitation
		• Skillful delivery of serious news
		Spiritual
		• Chaplain, social worker, or any clinician

(continued)

Table 1.2 Continued

Trajectory	Characteristics	Palliative Care Interventions for the Patient or Family[5,6,10,25,36-38]

4. Terminally ill and comes to the ED	• Patient, family, and primary provider achieve informal recognition and establish formal prognostication/certification that death is near (e.g., prognosis < 6 months enabling hospice enrollment).
	• Family nonetheless activates emergency medical system (e.g., calls 911) to bring patient to ED because of:
	  • Misunderstanding of the role of hospice
	  • Lack of experiential knowledge of signs of impending death
	  • Cultural/spiritual considerations.
		Physical/Symptoms
		• Pain and symptom medications
		• Consider withholding/withdrawing life-sustaining therapies and medicate for distressing symptoms
		Psychological & Social
		• Assess the reasons for coming to the ED
		• Clarify goals of care and match interventions to the goals of care
		• Assess for advance directives
		• Determine how decisions are made within the family (patient autonomy vs. shared decision-making)
		• Assess caregiver coping
		• Assess caregiver resource network and support
		• Family witnessed resuscitation
		• Skilful delivery of serious news
		Spiritual
		• Chaplain, social worker, or any clinician

5. Frail and hovering near death	• Patients are frail and critically ill and share many aspects with the terminally ill patient population (e.g., poor health/functional status). • ED clinicians, although uncertain, anticipate that the patient will die during this hospitalization. • No informal recognition or formal prognostication/certification that death is near (e.g., prognosis < 6 months).	Physical/Symptoms • Pain and symptom medications • Consider withholding/withdrawing life-sustaining therapies and medicate for distressing symptoms Psychological & Social • Assess the reasons for coming to the ED

	• Absence of this recognition or certification process causes ED clinicians to question the hopes and goals of the therapies that they initiate for the patient.	• Clarify goals of care and match interventions to the goals of care • Assess for advance directives • Determine how decisions are made within the family (patient autonomy vs. shared decision-making) • Assess caregiver coping • Assess caregiver resource network and support • Skillful delivery of serious news Spiritual • Chaplain, social worker, or any clinician
6. Alive and interactive on arrival, but arrests in the ED	• Death unexpected for both the clinicians and the family. • ED clinicians are surprised by the sudden death or arrest of the patient while they are in the process of trying to rule in or rule out life-threatening pathology or are actively trying to treat life-threatening pathology. • ED clinicians use all appropriate resources in an attempt to resuscitate the patient.	Physical/Symptoms • Pain and symptom medications Psychological & Social • Clarify goals of care and match interventions to the goals of care • Assess for advance directives • Determine how decisions are made within the family (patient autonomy vs. shared decision-making) • Family witnessed resuscitation • Skillful delivery of serious news Spiritual • Chaplain, social worker, or any clinician

(continued)

Table 1.2 Continued

Trajectory	Characteristics	Palliative Care Interventions for the Patient or Family[5,6,10,25,36-38]
7. Potentially preventable death by omission or commission	• The patient is approaching death and is dying, but this is not recognized until it is potentially too late. • Can occur in both routine and unfamiliar situations. • Index of suspicion of death or adverse event is not high and mistakes may be made. • ED clinicians' perceptions and what they choose to focus their attention on may lead them down the wrong evaluation or treatment pathway. • The clinicians forget guidelines for care, prioritize care for different patients differently, become desensitized to the care needs of the patient, or lack knowledge about how to deliver the best possible care.	Symptoms • Consider pain and symptom medications that will not interfere with hemodynamics (e.g., fentanyl) • Consider withholding/withdrawing life-sustaining therapies and medicate for distressing symptoms Psychological & Social • Clarification of goals of care and match interventions to the goals of care • Assess for advance directives • Determine how decisions are made within the family (patient autonomy vs. shared decision-making) • Family witnessed resuscitation • Skillful delivery of serious news and death ification Spiritual • Chaplain, social worker, or any clinician

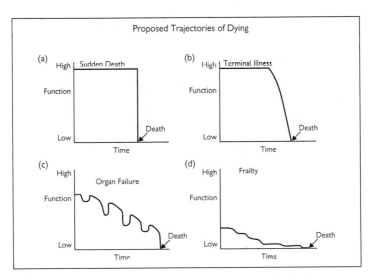

Figure 1.1 Theoretical Functional Trajectories of Dying. Reprinted with permission. Lunney JR, Lynn J, Hogan C. Profiles of older medicare decedents. J Am Geriatr Soc. 2002;50:1108–1112.

treated "baseline," and are likely to have a further decline after a given episode. For example, if we completely treat Mrs. X's exacerbation of her COPD, the best we could hope for would be her "usual" functional status.

It is also good to keep in mind that acute events can happen while a person is traversing along any dying trajectory. This has immense importance, and complications are the likely mode of death for patients with chronic illness. Many will choose to die at a particular time by refusing time-extending therapies when death is approaching, or when the time-extending therapies are too burdensome, or when the quality of life is too low.

Prognostication and Prognostic Tools

There are three reasons to identify and discuss prognosis in the ED when patients present with advanced illness or injury: (1) a decision about the kind of treatment given must be made in the ED; (2) the patient is at high risk of mortality during this hospitalization and if the patient wishes to tell family, they will likely benefit from knowing this information; and (3) the patient has a right to consider and refuse treatment that may prolong and increase his or her suffering, which includes disease-modifying treatment such as coronary stenting or resuscitation.

Emergency physicians are continually formulating and communicating prognosis. Because the hallmark of emergency medicine is timely evaluation, management, and disposition, we are constantly weighing how "good" or "bad" the condition is. We often tell the patient, "You have bronchitis and I think you will do 'just fine' at home with the following treatments." We are constantly weighing the chance of a fatal disease in a given patient. That said, prognosis is the least well-studied and discussed area in all of medicine, and there is little literature on communicating bad prognoses in emergency medicine. Nonetheless, the formulation and communication of a valid prognosis can be very helpful to patient, family, and physician colleagues alike.

Formulating and communicating a prognosis allows patients, families, and caregivers in the ED to evaluate the indications for treatment and to adjust expectations. Perhaps more than any other specialty, emergency medicine must on a daily basis use our best estimate of prognosis to break good or bad news, evaluate disposition, and consider appropriate utilization of resources.

The "surprise" question, "Would I be surprised if the patient died in the next 12 months?" has been a useful tool to identify patients with poor prognosis in primary care,[19] dialysis populations,[20,21] and outpatient oncology.[22] This question could also be used in patients with potentially life-limiting or life-threatening conditions in the hospital.[23] In the ED, we could reformulate the question to be, "Would I be surprised if the patient died in this hospitalization?" If the answer is yes, then the patient could benefit from palliative care interventions or specialists in this ED or hospitalization stay. Because the exact amount of time is unknown, it is helpful to consider time frames in terms of hours-to-days, days-to-weeks, weeks-to-months instead of giving specific time frames. The following selected prognostication tools may assist emergency clinicians in formulating prognoses:

Cancer

Cancer has many solid tumor and blood/lymph subtypes. Each cancer has unique trajectories. However, in advanced and widely metastatic cancer, there are some prognostic indicators that can help emergency clinicians understand whether the patient has days-to-weeks or weeks-to-months left to live.

The single most important factor for prognosis is functional ability.[24,25] Understanding the functional ability of patients with advanced cancer allows us to understand the activity and energy level. Two measures of functional ability are the Karnofsky Index[26] (Figure 1.2, 0 = dead, 100 = normal) and the Eastern Cooperative Oncology Group[27] ([ECOG] Figure 1.3; 0 = normal, 5 = dead). If a person spends $\geq$ 50% of the time confined to bed or chair (e.g., Karnofsky score of < 40% or ECOG > 3), the patient has a median survival of 3 months.[24] If there is significant symptom burden such as increased pain, dyspnea, or other symptoms, the survival time decreases.

Several cancer syndromes have well-documented short median times of survival (Table 1.3).[24,25]

Heart Failure

Two classification systems help categorize the severity of heart failure (HF). The New York Heart Association (NYHA) Functional Classification[28] (Table 1.4) provides a framework to assess the severity of HF based on the functional ability of the patient. The American College of Cardiology (ACC)/American Heart Association (AHA) Guidelines for Stages of Heart Failure[29] (Table 1.5) provide another method to classify the severity of HF. The ACC/AHA Guidelines are meant to supplement rather than replace the NYHA Functional Classification.

100% – normal, no complaints, no signs of disease
90% – capable of normal activity, few symptoms or signs of disease
80% – normal activity with some difficulty, some symptoms or signs
70% – caring for self, not capable of normal activity or work
60% – requiring some help, can take care of most personal requirements
50% – requires help often, requires frequent medical care
40% – disabled, requires special care and help
30% – severely disabled, hospital admission indicated but no risk of death
20% – very ill, urgently requiring admission, requires supportive measures or treatment
10% – moribund, rapidly progressive fatal disease processes
0% – death.

Figure 1.2 Karnofsky Performance Scale

0 – Asymptomatic (Fully active, able to carry on all pre-disease activities without restriction)
1 – Symptomatic but completely ambulatory (Restricted in physically strenuous activity but ambulatory and able to carry out work of a light or sedentary nature. For example, light housework, office work)
2 – Symptomatic, <50% In bed during the day (Ambulatory and capable of all self care but unable to carry out any work activities. Up and about more than 50% of waking hours)
3 – Symptomatic, >50% in bed, but not bedbound (Capable of only limited self-care, confined to bed or chair 50% or more of waking hours)
4 – Bedbound (Completely disabled. Cannot carry on any self-care. Totally confined to bed or chair)
5 – Death

Figure 1.3 Eastern Cooperative Oncology Group Performance Status

Table 1.3 Median Survival Times of Complications of Cancer

Cancer Complication	Median Survival Time
Multiple brain metastases (without radiation)	4–8 weeks
Multiple brain metastases (with radiation)	3–6 months
Malignant hypercalcemia (except newly diagnosed breast cancer, myeloma, or cancer responsive to cancer-directed therapy)	~8 weeks (i.e., weeks-to-months)
Malignant pericardial effusion	~8 weeks (i.e., weeks-to-months)
Carcinomatous meningitis	8–12 weeks
Malignant ascites, malignant pleural effusion, malignant bowel obstruction	< 6 months

Reprinted with permission. Emanuel L, Quest T, eds. The Education in Palliative and End-of-Life Care for Emergency Medicine. Chicago, IL: The EPEC™ Project; 2007.

Table 1.4 New York Heart Association Functional Classification[28]

Class 1	No limitation of physical activity. Ordinary physical activity does not cause undue fatigue or dyspnea.
Class 2	Slight limitation of physical activity. Comfortable at rest, but ordinary physical activity results in fatigue or dyspnea.
Class 3	Marked limitation of physical activity without symptoms. Symptoms are present even at rest. If any physical activity is undertaken, symptoms are increased.
Class 4	Unable to carry on any physical activity without symptoms. Symptoms are present even at rest. If any physical activity is undertaken, symptoms are increased.

Table 1.5 American College of Cardiology/American Heart Association Guidelines for Stages of Heart Failure[29]

A	Patients at high risk for heart failure because of the presence of conditions strongly associated with the development of heart failure. Such patients have no identified structural or functional abnormalities of the pericardium, myocardium, or cardiac valves and have never shown signs or symptoms of heart failure.
B	Patients who have structural heart disease that is strongly associated with the development of heart failure but who have never shown signs or symptoms of heart failure.
C	Patients who have current or prior symptoms of heart failure associated with underlying structural heart disease.
D	Patients with advanced structural heart disease and marked symptoms of heart failure at rest despite maximal medical therapy and who require specialized interventions.

Stages A and B describe those patients who are at risk of developing HF. Patients in Stages C or D should have the NYHA Functional Classification applied to determine severity of symptoms.

The Seattle Heart Failure Model[30] (www.SeattleHeartFailureModel.org) has been shown to be the most accurate tool in estimating the mean, 1-year, 2-year, and 5-year survival of patients with HF.[31]

Chronic Obstructive Pulmonary Disease

Chronic obstructive pulmonary disease (COPD) may be the most difficult disease to prognosticate. There are two staging systems for COPD: GOLD and BODE. GOLD (Global Initiative for Obstructive Lung Disease) is a staging system that is based on spirometry values of Forced Expiratory Volume in 1 second (FEV_1) and Forced Vital Capacity (FVC) as well as symptoms to determine the severity of the COPD (1 = mild, 4 = very severe).[32] The BODE (Body mass index/ airflow Obstruction/ Dyspnea/Exercise capacity) index has been validated as a tool for measuring disease severity and predicting survival.[33] Although these tools have been helpful in understanding the disease from a long-term perspective, the information needed to formulate a prognosis of either death or adverse event (e.g., exacerbation, hospitalization) often is not readily available to the emergency clinician. However, hypoxemia and hypercapnia are indicators of future adverse outcome or death.[34] Patients are eligible for hospice if the following criteria are met[25]:

- Dyspnea at rest
- Refractory to medical management with resultant decrease in functional capacity
- Oxygen saturation < 88%
- Frequent emergency department visits

It is important to discuss the hopes and goals of care in the setting of having these symptoms. Determining whether the patient has an advance directive or has discussed the concept of intubation is critical during this time of crisis in the ED.

Dementia

Dementia is a chronic, progressive, and incurable neurodegenerative disorder that can cause physical, psychological, social, and existential distress for patients and families.[25] Prognostication is difficult due to the slow indolent nature of the disease. Patients may have periods of plateaus and decline. In addition, patients do not die from their neurologic disease. Rather, they die as a result of the effects of impaired neurologic functioning on other body systems, such as a decrease in body weight due to anorexia. Often, patients die from an infectious process (e.g., pneumonia or sepsis). The National Hospice and Palliative Care Organization uses the following system to formulate a prognosis of ≤ 6 months:[25]

- Functional Assessment Staging (FAST) Stage 7C
- Need for assistance with at least three activities of daily living; increased frequency of bowel and bladder incontinence; inability to speak at least six intelligible words on an average day

Plus:

- Must have a history of one or more of the following in the last 12 months: aspiration, urinary tract infection, sepsis, pneumonia; multiple Stage III or IV pressure ulcers
- Evidence of nutritional compromise that includes an albumin of less than 2.5 or an unintentional weight loss of great than 10% over the last 12 months

Communicating the Prognosis

An important purpose for discussing prognosis is that it may affect the patient's actions, medical plan, and goals of care. If the information could not conceivably affect the patient's course of treatment or the patient's decisions about his life during the ED stay or the acute hospitalization, then there is no compelling reason to share prognostic information in the ED, unless the patient specifically asks for this. Clinicians also have many concerns about communicating prognoses; including fears that they may be wrong, the information may be upsetting to the patient or family, there may be conflict with the primary care provider, and there may be insufficient information to predict prognosis in an isolated encounter in the ED.

It is important to recognize that these median times are just numbers and that they do not help patients and families find meaning in the experience of coming to the ED in distress.[35] If possible, discussing the issues with the patient's primary care provider or specialist could be helpful in understanding what has been talked about and to co-create a plan of action. It is important to see this interaction as an opportunity to discuss the patient's hopes and goals for care in order to match resources and interventions with those hopes and goals. It is also an opportunity to dispel myths, such as unrealistic perceptions of success rates for cardiopulmonary resuscitation.

There are multiple ways to deliver the difficult news (see chapter 9). A core element of delivering the difficult or serious news is for the clinician to act as a guide in this unfamiliar territory for the patients and families and to ensure that they do not feel abandoned.

Creating a Plan of Action

Emergency clinicians can take the following steps in creating a plan of action:[25]

1. Identify the functional and the ED-specific trajectory given the patient's past medical history and current clinical presentation.
2. Formulate a prognosis based on the clinical data as well as other prognostic tools. Consider using the time frames of whether the patient will survive the hospitalization or the time frames of days, weeks, months, years rather than percentages of success rates or exact numbers.
3. Determine which interventions are appropriate given the patient's health status.
4. Elicit from the patient/family their understanding of the situation, their hopes, and their goals of care.
5. Deliver the difficult news in an interdisciplinary team of available personnel in the ED, such as the nurse, chaplain, or social worker.
6. Match the appropriate interventions and resources with the goals of care.
7. Communicate verbally and in writing with other healthcare team members as well as admitting services.
8. Ensure there is a smooth transition to the next service (home-based or inpatient care team).

Conclusion

Providing good emergency care is predicated on providing the best disease-modifying and palliative care possible. Our main goal should be to offer or provide only those interventions that are helpful and appropriate, and avoid those interventions that are nonbeneficial for patients and families. Understanding how patients approach death from both a functional and clinical trajectory and communicating a prognosis can inform how we set the path for patients and families as they move through the healthcare system.

References

1. Chan GK. End-of-life care models and emergency department care. *Acad Emerg Med*. 2004;11(1):79–86.

2. Smith AK, Fisher J, Schonberg MA, et al. Am I doing the right thing? Provider perspectives on improving palliative care in the emergency department. *Ann Emerg Med*. 2009;54(1):86–93, 93 e81.

3. Stone SC, Mohanty S, Grudzen CR, et al. Emergency medicine physicians' perspectives of providing palliative care in an emergency department. *J Palliat Med*. 2011;14(12):1333–1338.

4. Grudzen CR, Richardson LD, Hopper SS, Ortiz JM, Whang C, Morrison RS. Does palliative care have a future in the emergency department? Discussions with attending emergency physicians. *J Pain Symptom Manage*. 2012;43(1):1–9.

5. Heaston S, Beckstrand RL, Bond AE, Palmer SP. Emergency nurses' perceptions of obstacles and supportive behaviors in end-of-life care. *J Emerg Nurs*. 2006;32(6):477–485.

6. Beckstrand RL, Smith MD, Heaston S, Bond AE. Emergency nurses' perceptions of size, frequency, and magnitude of obstacles and supportive behaviors in end-of-life care. *J Emerg Nurs*. 2008;34(4):290–300.

7. Glaser BG, Strauss AL. *Time for Dying*. Chicago: Adline Publishing Company; 1968.

8. Field MJ, Cassel CK. *Approaching Death. Improving Care at the End of Life*. Washington, DC: Institute of Medicine; 1997.

9. Lunney JR, Lynn J, Hogan C. Profiles of older Medicare decedents. *JAGS*. 2002;50:1108–1112.

10. Emergency Nurses Association. End-of-Life Care in the Emergency Department. [Position Statement]. 2005; http://www.ena.org/SiteCollectionDocuments/Position%20Statements/End_of_Life_Care_in_the_Emergency_Department_-_ENA_PS.pdf. Accessed July 8, 2010.

11. Iserson KV. Withholding and withdrawing medical treatment: an emergency medicine perspective. *Ann Emerg Med*. 1996;28(1):51–54.

12. Marco CA, Bessman ES, Schoenfeld CN, Kelen GD. Ethical issues of cardiopulmonary resuscitation: current practice among emergency physicians. *Acad Emerg Med*. 1997;4(9):898–904.

13. Taylor JP, Taylor JE. Emergency nursing process and nursing diagnosis. In: Newberry L, ed. *Sheehy's Emergency Nursing: Principles and Practice*. 4th ed. St. Louis, MO: Mosby; 1998:9–15.

14. Kercher EE. Crisis intervention in the emergency department. *Emergency Medical Clinics of North America*. 1991;9(1):219–232.

15. Sanders AB. Unique aspects of ethics in emergency medicine. In: Iserson KV, Sanders AB, Mathieu D, eds. *Ethics in Emergency Medicine*. 2nd ed. Tuscon, AZ: Galen Press, Ltd.; 1995:7–10.

16. Walters DT, Tupin JP. Family grief in the emergency department. *Emergency Medical Clinics of North America*. 1991;9:189–207.

17. Bailey C, Murphy R, Porock D. Trajectories of end-of-life care in the emergency department. *Annals of Emergency Medicine*. 2011;57(4):362–369.

18. Chan GK. Trajectories of approaching death in the emergency department: clinician narratives of patient transitions to the end of life. *J Pain Symptom Manage*. 2011;42(6):864–881.

19. Pattison M, Romer AL. Improving Care Through the End of Life: launching a primary care clinic-based program. *J Palliat Med*. 2001;4(2):249–254.

20. Moss AH GJ, Sharma S, et al. Utility of the "surprise" question to identify dialysis patients with high mortality. *Clin J Am Soc Nephrol*. 2008;3:1379–1384.

21. Cohen LM RR, Moss AH, Germain MJ. Predicting six-month mortality for patients who are on maintenance hemodialysis. *Clin J Am Soc Nephrol*. 2010;5:72–79.

22. Moss AH, Lunney JR, Culp S, et al. Prognostic significance of the "surprise" question in cancer patients. *J Palliat Med*. 2010;13(7):837–840.

23. Weissman DE, Meier DE. Identifying patients in need of a palliative care assessment in the hospital setting: a consensus report from the Center to Advance Palliative Care. *J Palliat Med*. 2011;14(1):17–23.

24. Weissman DE. Fast Facts #13: Determining prognosis in advanced cancer. 2009. http://www.eperc.mcw.edu/fastfact/ff_013.htm. Accessed March 25, 2012.

25. Emanuel L, Quest T, eds. *The Education in Palliative and End-of-Life Care for Emergency Medicine*. Chicago, IL: The EPEC™ Project; 2007.

26. Karnofsky D, Burchenal J. The clinical evaluation of chemotherapeutic agents in cancer. In: Macleod C, ed. *Evaluation of Chemotherapeutic Agents*. New York, NY: Columbia University Press; 1949:191–205.

27. Oken MM, Creech RH, Tormey DC, et al. Toxicity and response criteria of the Eastern Cooperative Oncology Group. *Am J Clin Oncol*. 1982;5:649–655.

28. The Criteria Committee of the New York Heart Association. *Nomenclature and Criteria for Diagnosis of Diseases of the Heart and Great Vessels*. 9th ed. Boston: Little, Brown; 1994.

29. Hunt SA, Abraham WT, Chin MH, et al. 2009 Focused update incorporated into the ACC/AHA 2005 Guidelines for the Diagnosis and Management of Heart Failure in Adults. A Report of the American College of Cardiology Foundation/ American Heart Association Task Force on Practice Guidelines Developed in Collaboration With the International Society for Heart and Lung Transplantation. *J Am Coll Cardiol*. 2009;53(15):e1–e90.

30. Levy WC, Mozaffarian D, Linker DT, et al. The Seattle Heart Failure Model: prediction of survival in heart failure. *Circulation*. 2006;113(11):1424–1433.

31. Nakayama M, Osaki S, Shimokawa H. Validation of mortality risk stratification models for cardiovascular disease. *Am J Cardiol*. 2011;108(3):391–396.

32. Rabe KF, Hurd S, Anzueto A, et al. Global strategy for the diagnosis, management, and prevention of chronic obstructive pulmonary disease: GOLD executive summary. *Am J Respir Crit Care Med*. 2007;176(6):532–555.

33. Celli BR, Cote CG, Marin JM, et al. The body-mass index, airflow obstruction, dyspnea, and exercise capacity index in chronic obstructive pulmonary disease. *N Engl J Med*. 2004;350(10):1005–1012.

34. Matkovic Z, Huerta A, Soler N, et al. Predictors of adverse outcome in patients hospitalised for exacerbation of chronic obstructive pulmonary disease. *Respiration*. 2012; 84(1):17–26.

35. Gould SJ. The median isn't the message. 2002. http://cancerguide.org/median_not_msg.html. Accessed March 20, 2012.

36. Clarke R. Improving end-of-life care in emergency departments. *Emerg Nurse*. 2008;16(7):34–37.

37. Norton CK, Hobson G, Kulm E. Palliative and end-of-life care in the emergency department: Guidelines for nurses. *J Emerg Nurs*. 2011;37(3)240–245.

38. Ferrell BR, Dahlin C, Campbell ML, Paice JA, Malloy P, Virani R. End-of-life nursing education consortium (ELNEC) training program: Improving palliative care in critical care. *Crit Care Nurs Q*. 2007;30(3):206–212.

Chapter 2

Rapid Palliative Care Assessment

Eric Bryant, MD, FACEP

Introduction

Emergency clinicians are continually clarifying goals and expectations of patients and families. Why did you come to the emergency department (ED) today? What are you expecting we might do for you? This becomes more of a challenge when patients have serious life-threatening illness. An uncomfortable tension can develop in the busy, distracting environment of the ED; is it the right environment to consider alternatives to life-sustaining therapies (such as comfort care) or alternative dispositions to acute hospitalization in severely ill patients (such as home with hospice services)? In the absence of information, it is the ethical and legal obligation of emergency clinicians to institute life-prolonging therapies in serious illness. However, if information is available or could be obtained, in the spirit of informed consent, it is the obligation of the emergency clinician to assess what the patient/surrogate is hoping for and expecting, and to base interventions on the patient's values and goals. The presumption that all patients present to the ED because they want life-threatening conditions identified and treated, and always want their lives prolonged, is overly simplistic and outdated.

The life-saving imperative is rooted in emergency medicine training, practice, reimbursement, and medical-legal risk avoidance. Nevertheless, there is a growing recognition that many patients present for reasons other than life prolongation, such as the presence of severe, uncontrolled symptoms; unsafe living conditions; and family/caregiver conflict or distress. Emergency clinicians are under pressure to deliver the highest quality care in the least amount of time. However, the failure to recognize significant social, psychological, or spiritual contributors to suffering can easily lead to unnecessary and potentially harmful testing, suboptimal resource utilization to provide needed care (such as an undesired admission to the intensive care unit), and patient/family dissatisfaction. As with other patients in the ED, some element of triage should occur. The emergency clinician can use a team approach to assess social, psychological, or spiritual contributors. Elements examined in patients who are unstable may differ from those examined in patients who have been stabilized. This chapter will focus on rapid palliative care assessment of patients who present to the ED in the context of their clinical presentation (Figure 2.1).

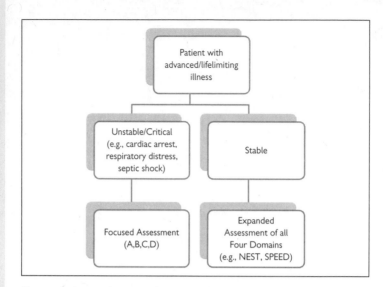

Figure 2.1 Assessment: unstable versus stable patient

The Critically Ill or Unstable Patient

When a patient is unstable and will die without rapid airway protection, breathing support, arrhythmia control, or blood pressure support, time is very limited. Many patients with chronic advanced illness present to the emergency department critically ill. Although sepsis, respiratory failure, and mental-status changes are often signs of a new and acute injury or illness, they also can be part of the common final pathway of a chronic progressive illness such as dementia, congestive heart failure (CHF), chronic obstructive pulmonary disease (COPD), and metastatic cancer. The default setting in emergency medicine is to resuscitate and stabilize first. This places patients who are critically ill on an intensive pathway from the beginning of their hospitalization, regardless of their goals or wishes in seeking care in the ED. However, within the limitations of time and acuity every effort should be made to perform a focused assessment and clarify the goals of emergency care, even for an unstable patient. A quick visual inspection may inform the assessment immediately, a few words from emergency medical services (EMS) or the knowledge that the patient is presenting from a nursing facility also can offer a quick clue that a patient is chronically ill. When an actively dying patient comes to the ED due to uncontrolled symptoms, are they seeking to reverse the dying process with hope of recovery or are they seeking comfort? While this is being clarified, there are key palliative care elements to consider.

In the unstable patient, emergency providers are trained to follow the ABCs of resuscitation: airway, breathing, circulation, and in trauma—disability. A parallel ABCD assessment of four critical elements of a rapid palliative care model

---

The ABCD Assessment

Is there an **A**dvance care plan or advance directive?

Can there be **B**etter symptom control?

Who are the key **C**aregivers?

Does the patient have **D**ecisional capacity?

Figure 2.2 The ABCD Assessment of Immediate Palliative Care Needs in Unstable Patients

includes the following questions: Is there an *Advance care plan?* Can we make the symptoms *Better?* Is there a *Caregiver/surrogate?* And does the patient have *Decision-making capacity?* (Figure 2.2) This assessment should be done with the ED interdisciplinary team working together (physician, nurse, liaison/advocate, social worker, and chaplain) to clarify key issues and improve the likelihood that treatment will be consistent with goals of care. In addition, family presence at the bedside in the initial treatment of a critically ill patient, while potentially challenging for the treatment team may be of great benefit. In fact, the presence of family may help in determining the appropriateness of initiating or withholding invasive life-prolonging measures or discontinuing unwanted or nonbeneficial interventions.

These questions can be asked by any member of the care team, even as initial resuscitation efforts proceed. One of the advantages of having an appropriate surrogate member present during initial assessment and stabilization of a patient is that it can facilitate a concurrent approach. Although the assessment is presented here in alphabetical order, in practice one would start with "D": Is the patient decisional? A patient who is alert and cognitively intact should be guiding their own care. In the setting of hemodynamic instability or out-of-control symptoms, such as pain or dyspnea, a patient may not be able to make complex medical decisions but can still often express basic preferences and contribute to decision-making with other family or caregivers. If the patient is not decisional, is there a written advance directive or otherwise known care plan that expresses the patient's wishes? Patients' may not have executed a formal directive, yet they may have expressed their wishes to their surrogates. Among other things, a directive may indicate who patients want to make medical decisions if they are unable to do so themselves. Advance directives often give some guidance on resuscitation and life-prolonging therapies, although many "living will" documents address only prolonged life support in the setting of brain injury. Whether a designated medical durable power of attorney or other formally identified proxy is available, caregivers and family members can provide important information about patients, including their baseline condition and their wishes. Family members and caregivers may also experience disagreement or distress, and their needs will need to be anticipated and addressed. While the issues of decision-making and care preferences are being sorted out, it is important to treat the patient's symptoms. In addition to relieving the patient's suffering and the family's distress, symptom management can often improve a patient's cognition and ability to participate in decision-making.

The Medically Stable Patient

If a patient is stable at the time of presentation, or stabilizes in the course of treatment, then a deeper assessment of palliative care needs can take place. An exhaustive assessment of all four domains is not usually practical in an ED encounter, but the process can begin in the ED. It may involve different members of the care team over the course of the ED stay and beyond. The key is to recognize the importance of all four domains (physical, psychological, social, and spiritual), and to have a standardized approach to initiating the conversation, as well as a means to document information so the process can be continued by the admitting team or outpatient provider, depending on the patient's disposition. Identifying palliative care needs in the ED for patients who are not critically ill or actively dying is important for several reasons:

1. Many ED patients are discharged to home or a higher level of care, such as an assisted living facility, skilled nursing facility, or long-term care facility, precluding an inpatient assessment.
2. Identifying needs prior to discharge can lead to better coordination with outside services and reduce return visits.
3. Patients with advanced illness and limited prognosis are often eligible for hospice care and may prefer to enroll in hospice rather than be admitted to the hospital.

For patients being admitted to the hospital, an extended palliative care assessment can take place after admission. However, clarifying and documenting patient goals and needs at the outset of the admission can help focus treatment, trigger early involvement of palliative care specialists, and document treatment preferences regarding resuscitation or artificial nutrition or hydration (ANH). The latter is particularly important if the patient were to decline suddenly after admission.

Use of a Structured Approach

One structured approach to palliative care assessment is known as the Needs at the End-of-life Screening Tool (NEST). Based on work by Emanuel and colleagues, NEST stands for Needs, Existential, Symptoms, and Therapeutic—a reframing of the four domains discussed previously. (Figure 2.3) The mnemonic can be useful for remembering the components but does not need to direct the order in which issues are addressed. In the ED it often appropriate to begin with Symptoms and Therapeutics.

Points to Remember

1. Missing one of the domains over the course of an assessment can leave a significant source of suffering unaddressed. This can result in ambivalence or disagreement about goals, dissatisfaction with care, or repeat ED visits for vague or chronic complaints.
2. It is neither realistic nor necessary for one provider to perform a complete assessment covering all domains. All ED team members should be supported in contributing to the overall assessment.

The NEST Assessment*

***Performed by the ED Interdisciplinary Team**

- Are there social **N**eeds (including financial and caregiver issues) that should guide patient disposition?
- Does the patient have **E**xistential needs (around meaning/spiritual/faith/forgiveness) that contribute to distress?
- What physical or mental **S**ymptoms led to this ED visit and require treatment?
- What should the **T**herapeutic goals be for this ED visit or hospitalization?

Needs	1. How much of a financial hardship is your illness for you or your family?
	2. How much trouble do you have accessing the medical care you need?
	3. How often is there someone to confide in?
	4. How much help do you need with things like getting meals or getting to the doctor?
Existential	1. How much does this illness seem senseless and meaningless?
	2. How much does religious belief or your spiritual life contribute to your sense of purpose?
	3. How much have you settled your relationship with the people close to you?
	4. Since your illness, how much do you live your life with a special sense of purpose?
Symptom matters	1. How much do you suffer from physical symptoms such as pain, shortness of breath, fatigue, bowel or urinary problems?
	2. How often do you feel confused or anxious or depressed?
Therapeutic	1. How much do you feel your doctors and nurses respect you as an individual?
	2. How clear is the information from the medical team about what to expect regarding your illness?
	3. How much do you feel that the medical care you are getting fits with your goals?

Figure 2.3 The NEST Assessment for Palliative Care Needs

3. A pocket card or embedding a template in a preformatted chart or electronic record can prompt all staff to attend to and record information relevant to the assessment.
4. Like any procedure or intervention, a palliative care assessment requires training and practice.

Summary

Although time and space constraints, as well as patient acuity, can place significant limits on a palliative care assessment in the ED, it remains the responsibility of the ED provider to ensure that the treatment a patient receives is in alignment with patient goals, including whether to receive intensive life-prolonging measures or to receive intensive comfort care. A brief, focused assessment can be conducted concurrently with initial stabilization efforts to determine whether the default resuscitation and life-support measures are, in fact, consistent with the patient's wishes, or if a focus on or transition to a comfort approach is desired. The ED provider should be able to manage symptoms and provide support for a patient and family, especially when death is the expected outcome. For stable patients who have an advanced illness, the ED is an important setting to assess for unmet palliative care needs, initiate a discussion about goals of care, and document in a way that allows subsequent providers to continue the conversation.

With the development of numerous life-prolonging interventions in the last century a dichotomy has grown between curative intent and providing comfort. Many interventions cause increased discomfort, but this is felt to be offset by the improvement in long-term survival. This dichotomy has had the unfortunate consequence of viewing treatments as "all or nothing" with a perceived line between life-prolonging treatments and end-of-life care, only crossed when a patient enrolls in hospice. In fact, patients may have multiple and even seemingly contradictory goals. The challenge for emergency providers is not to fixate on which side of the "line" a patient is on, but rather to recognize where they are on the trajectory of their illness, to understand the tradeoffs involved in pursuing or declining certain treatments, and to help a patient communicate priorities. This gradual shift in goals is common and seems intuitive, but it would be wrong to make assumptions about any particular patient's wishes without asking. While emergency providers may be unfamiliar with asking about goals of care, patients and families are often inexperienced at being asked. It is useful to have a basic framework for palliative care assessment that can be worked into a brief ED history and physical exam and incorporate the expertise of the entire ED team.

References

1. Emanuel L, Alpert H, Emanuel E. Concise screening questions for clinical assessments of terminal care: the needs near the end-of-life care screening tool. *J Palliat Med.* 2001;4(4):465–474.

2. Education in Palliative and End of Life Care (EPEC). *EPEC for Emergency Medicine.* Rapid Palliative Care Assessment. 2008. Available at: http://epec.net/epec_em.php Accessed July 7, 2012.

Chapter 3

Cancer Emergencies

Jessica Stetz, MD, MS and Audrey Tan, DO

Introduction

Malignancies often cause distressing symptoms that may require emergent interventions. Metastatic spinal cord compression (MSCC), superior vena cava syndrome (SVCS), and malignant hypercalcemia are three important syndromes that emergency physicians must recognize and manage well.

Spinal Cord Compression

The spine is the most common site for metastatic disease and spinal cord compression is a common complication. In addition to causing significant pain, it may also result in a devastating loss of neurologic function and increased mortality. The median survival for spinal metastasis is approximately 10 months overall, but in those with spinal cord compression, median survival decreases to approximately 3 months. Additionally, the preservation of function toward the end of life is a universally important goal. Patients who become bed-bound lose independence and experience a profound alteration in self-image.

Pathophysiology

Metastatic spinal cord compression may be defined as the compression of the dural sac, spinal cord, or cauda equina by an extradural tumor or associated edema. It is diagnosed radiographically by the indentation of the theca at the level of clinical signs and symptoms.[1]

When the bony or adjacent structures of the spine are infiltrated with malignancy, the spinal cord becomes vulnerable to compression and injury. The spinal canal is composed of the vertebral body anteriorly, the spinous process posteriorly, with the lamina and pedicles laterally completing the ring. Within the bony ring is the thecal sac, with the dura as the outermost layer. Metastatic spinal cord compression occurs when tumor or edema compresses the thecal sac, leading to compression of spinal nervous tissue within the dura, causing pain, ischemia, and neurologic compromise. Metastatic spinal cord compression is primarily caused by vasogenic edema from adjacent metastases, rather than direct tumor invasion.

Epidemiology

More than 20,000 U.S. cancer patients a year develop symptomatic MSCC.[2] The development of MSCC is more commonly associated with certain malignancies.

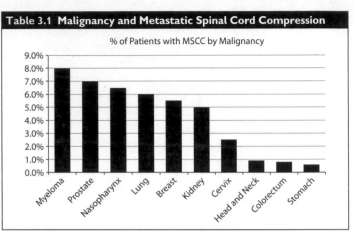

Table 3.1 **Malignancy and Metastatic Spinal Cord Compression**

% of Patients with MSCC by Malignancy

Loblaw DA, Lapierre NJ, Mackillop WJ. A population-based study of malignant spinal cord compression in Ontario. *Clin Oncol.* 2003;15(4):211–217.

In adults, these malignancies are prostate, lung, breast, multiple myeloma, nasopharyngeal, and kidney.[5] In the pediatric population, the tumors that most commonly lead to MSCC are sarcomas and neuroblastomas, followed by germ cell tumors and lymphomas.[4] Table 3.1 summarizes the tumors that most commonly cause MSCC.

Signs and Symptoms

Pain is usually the first symptom of MSCC. A vast majority of patients with MSCC present with back pain that is often referred and poorly localized. Historically, 60%–85% of patients have been unable to ambulate at the time of diagnosis, but more recent statistics suggest that earlier diagnosis of MSCC is increasing.[6,7,8] Delayed presentation is associated with poorer functional outcomes in terms of gait, mobility, and continence.[7] The best predictor of post-treatment neurologic outcome is pretreatment functional ability. Expeditious diagnosis preserves neurologic function and is more successful than attempting to reverse established deficits.

Diagnosis

Clinicians must have a high index of suspicion for MSCC in any cancer patient presenting with new or changed back pain. Magnetic resonance imaging (MRI) is the gold standard for diagnosis of MSCC. Magnetic resonance imaging of the entire spine is recommended because the radiation field may be altered in up to 40% of patients by unexpected findings.[9] If MRI is not feasible due to contraindications or inaccessibility, computed tomography (CT) myelography is the next-best diagnostic option. A majority of lesions causing MSCC occur in the thoracic spine (60%–70%), 20%–30% in the lumbosacral spine, and 10% in the cervical region.[5]

Interventions

Goals of care must be addressed at each step and the burden of each therapy weighed against the likelihood of benefit. Pain and symptom management must be aggressive. Analgesia will often be required to perform a physical examination and is nearly always necessary for the prolonged positioning required for imaging. Acute pain is best addressed with parenteral opioids. In the longer term, oral medications and adjuvants may be useful. Anxiety, depression, and changes in self-image are common and best managed by a multidisciplinary team. Constipation must be considered in any patient who is immobilized or placed on opioids. In MSCC, both autonomic dysfunction and opioid use may exacerbate constipation.

A 2008 Cochrane review assessed the benefits and harms of interventions utilized in the treatment of MSCC, specifically corticosteroids, radiation therapy (RT), and surgery, as well as ambulation and survival data.[10]

Corticosteroids

Three small trials with a combined sample size of 105 patients did not show significant benefit from corticosteroid administration. Three groups were compared (high-dose dexamethasone [96–100 mg], versus moderate-dose [10–16 mg], versus no dose) in terms of ambulation, two-year survival, analgesia, and urinary incontinence.[11,12,13] Higher doses were associated with a significant increase in serious adverse outcomes, such as perforated gastric ulcer, psychosis, and infectious deaths, as well as undesirable effects such as anxiety, tremulousness, and altered mental status. Despite a dearth of evidence, corticosteroid administration remains the de facto standard of care. It is likely that steroids will continue to be used in the management of MSCC although high-dose steroids should be used with caution.

Radiation Therapy

Radiation therapy (RT) is the most common intervention in MSCC. Various dosing schedules have been employed, commonly multi-fraction therapy 30 Gray (Gy) in 10 fractions (ranging from 20 to 40 Gy). Alternatively, some patients receive a single fraction of 8 to 10 Gy. In 2005, Marranzano compared different RT doses and schedules on patients with poor prognoses. There was no difference in analgesia, ambulation, recurrence, survival, or toxicity between patients receiving 16 Gy in two fractions or 30 Gy in eight.[14] More recently, Rades reported that a longer course of therapy is associated with improved local tumor control albeit similar analgesic and survival rates.[15]

According to a 2008 Cochrane review of single fraction versus multi-fraction RT for metastatic bone pain, approximately 60% of patients experienced significant pain relief after RT.[16] Analgesia was similar in multi-fraction and single-fraction therapy, although patients who had a single fraction required more retreatment than patients who had multi-fraction therapy (21% vs 7%) and experienced almost twice as many fractures (3% vs 1.6%).[16] Based on the data, single fraction therapy may be more appropriate for patients with a shorter life expectancy, as it limits the time spent in treatment, thereby improving quality of life and limiting costs.

Intensity modulated radiation therapy (IMRT) is high-precision radiotherapy that uses computer-controlled linear accelerators to deliver precise doses of radiation directly to the tumor. Intensity modulated radiation therapy allows the radiation dose to conform to the three-dimensional shape of the tumor by modulating the intensity of the radiation beam into multiple small volumes.

Intensity modulated radiation therapy maximizes radiation dose while minimizing toxicity. Very limited data is available on the efficacy of IMRT in MSCC. At this time, IMRT is available only at specialized centers.

Surgery

An early study published in 1980 on laminectomies was aborted secondary to increased harm.[17] With the advent of newer surgical techniques, a 2005 meta-analysis of nonrandomized RT versus surgical case-series suggested improved rates of ambulation following surgical intervention, particularly in patients who had recently lost the ability to walk.[18] Shortly thereafter, a randomized, controlled trial by Patchell showed significant benefit from surgery in a highly selected subset of patients.[2] The patients had a prognosis of at least three months, histologic diagnosis of cancer that was nonradiosensitive, MRI evidence of MSCC restricted to a single area, at least one sign of neurological compromise, including pain, and if paraplegic, had been so for less than 48 hours. In this group of 101 subjects, immediate decompressive surgery with resection and spinal stabilization significantly improved neurologic function, specifically ambulation. More patients could walk after surgery plus RT, than after RT alone (84% vs. 57%), and those patients retained the ability to walk for longer (122 days vs. 13 days). Significantly more paraplegic patients in the surgical group regained the ability to walk (10/16 vs. 3/16). Survival benefit was small but significant. Surgical patients lived on average 126 days compared to patients who received RT alone (100 days). The need for steroids and opioid analgesia was less in the surgical group. The study was stopped early once a predetermined early stopping criterion was fulfilled. In this landmark study, a select group of higher functioning patients benefited from surgery over conventional RT.

A 2009 randomized trial evaluated the effect of age on outcome in patients who underwent RT and surgery versus RT alone. The results demonstrated that increasing age appears to decrease the benefit of surgical intervention versus RT. Patients younger than 65 years appear to benefit from surgical intervention plus RT while patients older than 65 years did not appear to benefit from the addition of surgery.[19]

In 2010, Rades published a matched-pair analysis comparing surgery to RT, in a less selective, more representative group of patients with MSCC, than the patients in the Patchell study. Outcomes were equivalent in the surgery and the RT groups vis-à-vis improvement in motor function, ambulation, and one-year survival, suggesting that surgery is not beneficial for the majority of patients who experience MSCC.[8] Further research is warranted to determine the appropriate patient population with MSCC for whom surgical intervention would be beneficial.

Bisphosphonates

Bisphosphonates have been shown to decrease morbidity from metastatic disease in breast cancer and multiple myeloma. They are now used prophylactically in the management of newly diagnosed myeloma and in breast cancer patients with early metastases to prevent the progression of bony metastases. Bisphosphonates also decrease pain from bony metastatic disease and can be used as an adjunctive pain strategy.[20] Their role in the prevention and management of MSCC requires further investigation.

Prognosis

The most important prognostic indicator of post-treatment ambulation is the ability to ambulate at the time of diagnosis. The speed at which the primary tumor metastasizes also predicts survival.[6] Prognosis of MSCC is dependent on that of the underlying malignancy. Specifically, myeloma and breast cancer patients survive approximately five to six months whereas lung cancer patients survive one month. With intervention, survival of MSCC is approximately three months whereas without intervention, survival is one month.[3]

In summary, MSCC is a common, painful condition that may cause a catastrophic loss of mobility. Aggressive pain and symptom management is crucial. Suspicion must be high and imaging must be expeditious. High-dose steroids are associated with significantly more adverse effects and should be used with caution, although moderate-dose glucocorticoids are still thought to be beneficial despite limited evidence. Radiation therapy improves pain in the majority of patients with MSCC and single-fraction dosing should be considered in patients with a limited life expectancy. Neurosurgery may improve neurological outcome and quality of life in selected patients.

Superior Vena Cava Syndrome

Superior vena cava syndrome (SVCS) is the obstruction of blood through the superior vena cava (SVC) to the right atrium. It is most often a manifestation of malignancy, most typically lung, and can progress to the point of requiring emergent interventions. It is important to recognize the range of presentations, understand proper assessment and initiate timely interventions to avoid unnecessary morbidity.

Pathophysiology

The SVC is the major vessel collecting venous return to the heart from the head, arms, and upper torso. The left and right brachiocephalic veins join to form the SVC, which then extends caudally for 6 to 8 cm, travelling anterior to the right mainstem bronchus and terminating in the superior right atrium. The SVC is joined posteriorly by the azygos vein, which lies to the right of the ascending aorta. The mediastinal parietal pleura is lateral to the SVC, and the right paratracheal, azygos, right hilar, and subcarinal lymph node groups are adjacent to it. In this confined space, this thin-walled, low-pressure vessel is highly susceptible to compression and obstruction.

Three common pathologic mechanisms lead to SVCS.[21] The first is compromised vessel anatomy via extrinsic compression from a mass in the middle or anterior mediastinum, generally originating from a tumor of the right upper lobe bronchus. Alternatively, right paratracheal or precarinal lymph nodes may also compress the SVC as lung cancer generally spreads via the lymphatic system. The second mechanism is compromised venous flow, typically resulting from an occlusive or near-occlusive venous thrombus. The third mechanism is compromised vessel wall integrity, most often due to the presence of an intravascular device such as the tip of an indwelling catheter or a lead. Pathologic mechanisms often coexist resulting in an obstruction that is multifactorial, such as a patient with a mediastinal tumor and a hypercoagulable state, or a child with lymphoma who also has an indwelling central line.[21]

Obstruction of the SVC leads to increasing resistance to venous flow causing the diversion of blood through collateral veins. These collaterals assist in both diverting venous return and partially relieving the upper body of passive fluid congestion, particularly in chronic presentations.

The severity of the presentation of SVCS is variable. SVCS is clinically more severe if the obstruction is below the level of the azygos vein, underscoring the importance of this vessel for collateral circulation. The acuity of the obstruction also dictates severity, as collateral vessels require several weeks in order to dilate sufficiently to accommodate diverted blood. Finally, the degree of obstruction has a significant impact on the patient's symptomatology.

Etiology

In the early 20th century, infections, including syphilis and mediastinitis secondary to tuberculosis, accounted for a large proportion of SVC syndrome.[21] Since the advent of antibiotics, infectious causes of SVC syndrome have decreased dramatically.

Currently, SVCS is most commonly a complication of malignancy, leading to approximately 90% of cases.[22,23] Specifically, it is most frequently associated with lung cancer and lymphoma. Superior vena cava syndrome occurs in 2%–4% of all patients with lung cancer with a higher incidence in small cell lung cancer (SCLC) (incidence of approximately 10%)[22,24] and approximately 2% in non-small cell lung cancer (NSCLC).[24] In patients with lymphoma, SVCS occurs in 2%–4% of non-Hodgkins lymphoma, but despite mediastinal lymphadenopathy, it is relatively rare in Hodgkin's lymphoma.[22] Less common causes include metastatic disease and intrathoracic tumors such as mesotheliomas and thymomas.[23]

Nonmalignant causes of SVCS comprise approximately 10% of cases and include fibrosing mediastinitis and thrombosis of indwelling intravascular devices and/or pacemaker leads.[22]

Signs and Symptoms

The most common symptoms of SVCS include facial or neck swelling (82%), which is exacerbated by bending over or lying down; arm swelling (68%); dyspnea (66%); cough (50%); and dilated chest veins (38%).[22] Physicians should be aware that the presence of a headache, blurry vision, or nausea may represent early signs of cerebral edema, whereas confusion or obtundation suggest later presentation.[21,25,26] Similarly, stridor or airway compromise are signs of laryngeal edema and significant obstruction.

Diagnosis

The diagnosis of SVCS begins with a thorough physical exam. The extent of facial, neck, and/or arm swelling should be noted as well as the presence of collateral veins on the chest. Respiratory compromise should trigger increased concern and the patient's mental status should be noted.

Imaging plays a central role in determining pathologic mechanisms and guiding management. A chest radiograph is generally the first step in diagnostic imaging. An abnormality is noted in 78% of patients. The most common findings include mediastinal widening (64%) and pleural effusions (26%).[22]

A computed tomography (CT)scan of the chest with intravenous contrast is generally the most useful imaging modality. It allows the level and extent of obstruction to be visualized, evaluation of collateral pathways, identification of an intravascular thrombus, and provides information as to the etiology of the obstruction.[22,23] Magnetic resonance imaging (MRI) may be utilized for those patients with contraindications to CT scan. The presence of dilated collateral vessels on CT or MRI is highly suggestive of SVCS, with a sensitivity of 96% and specificity of 92%.[27]

Venography is generally reserved for cases in which prior imaging is inconclusive or an interventional stent is planned.

Interventions

Treatment is dictated by the severity of symptoms, likelihood of response to a particular treatment, the treatment of the malignancy itself, and the patient's goals for treatment. Supportive measures may provide symptomatic relief with minimal risk. Oxygen support and efforts to minimize hydrostatic pressure in the upper torso by fluid restriction and head elevation are recommended. Diuretics are often given, although there is little evidence supporting use.[22] Steroids are a temporizing measure used to reduce edema and associated symptoms, although there is no data documenting efficacy.[22] If utilized, steroid administration should be brief; chronic use can worsen facial swelling and may lead to fluid retention, both of which may worsen SVCS.[22]

No evidence exists to support routine anticoagulation in patients with SVCS without thrombosis,[22] although in the absence of substantial risk, many advocate for empiric anticoagulation given that most presentations involve thrombus formation and propagation.[21]

Radiation Therapy and Chemotherapy

If the obstruction of the SVC is caused by a malignancy known to be unresponsive to chemotherapy, radiotherapy can be offered. Radiotherapy is effective in providing relief in 75% of patients with SVCS due to SCLC and 66% of patients with SVCS due to NSCLC.[22] However, the recurrence rate is as high as 33%.[28] Complications include esophagitis, weight loss, skin irritation, and initial worsening of symptoms secondary to edema.[28] Radiotherapy is considered most appropriate as single therapy for NSCLC, and it may be used alone or as part of combination therapy in the treatment of patients with SCLC or lymphoma.[28]

Chemotherapy is an option for sensitive tumors such as lymphomas, SCLCs, and germ cell tumors. Response rates are highest in SCLCs (approximately 60%).[22] Although synchronous chemoradiation is an option, the data suggest that the relief of SVC symptoms is nearly equal for SCLC patients treated with either chemotherapy (77%) or radiation therapy (78%), or both chemotherapy and radiotherapy (83%).[25] Chemotherapy and radiation are not as effective for NSCLC-related SVCS. Reported response rates for relief of SVC obstruction in NSCLC are 59% (chemotherapy), 63% (radiation therapy), and 31% for synchronous chemoradiation.[25] Disadvantages of chemotherapy include the side effects of individual antineoplastic agents and prolonged onset of relief, which generally ranges from 2 to 4 weeks.[29,30]

Endovascular Stenting

Endovascular stenting is currently the treatment of choice for SVCS. Stent place-ment was previously used only adjunctively with radiotherapy or chemotherapy or for recurrence following conventional treatment.[29] In the past decade, it has been suggested that stents be considered first-line intervention in patients with malignant SVCS because stenting does not interfere with subsequent antitumor regimens and provides urgent relief of symptoms, thereby improving quality of life with few complications.[24,25,27,29]

Stenting occurs angiographically with the introduction of a guide wire via either subclavian or internal jugular vein with or without balloon angioplasty, followed by the deployment of a stent.[22] If a clot is encountered, thrombolytics may be considered. Morbidity does appear to be higher with the use of throm-bolytics.[22,23] Proponents advocate for clot lysis or thrombectomy to relieve symptoms, better elucidate the morphology of the lesion, and permit optimal stenting or angioplasty.[28]

Overall response rates of 95% with stent insertion are reported from a vari-ety of case series and systematic reviews, with an 11% recurrence rate.[23,24,25,30] The long-term patency rate was 92%.[21,13]

Following a stenting procedure, disease recurrence may be due to in-stent thrombosis, restenosis, or tumor ingrowth and may require secondary endo-vascular intervention.[21] Despite the lack of data, most patients are started on anticoagulation or antiplatelet therapy for variable durations.[21] Poststenting complications (0%–19%), include SVC rupture, hemorrhage, hemoptysis, epistaxis, pericardial tamponade, cardiac failure, recurrent laryngeal palsy, stent migration, pulmonary emboli, and groin hematoma.[24,28]

Surgery is the last resort for patients with SVCS, although rarely an option, as the tumor is often not resectable and patients are poor surgical candidates due to advanced disease and poor prognosis.[22] Surgery is reserved for cases not amenable to or that have failed endovascular intervention.[21] Bypass is usually performed from a patent vein above the level of obstruction (e.g., jugular or innominate) to the right atrium through a median sternotomy incision.[28]

The advantages and disadvantages of chemotherapy, radiation therapy and endovascular stent placement are summarized in Table 3.2.

Prognosis

Although heavily dependent on the underlying malignant condition, the median life expectancy in patients with SVCS is approximately 6 months with a range of 1.5 to 9.5 months.[21,26,30] Interestingly, in numerous reports of patients achiev-ing long-term (>5 yrs) survival, it appears to be equivalent to survival statistics of patients with same tumor type and stage without SVCS. This highlights the importance of aggressive symptom management.

In summary, SVCS is a disease process that has a marked impact on quality of life. Generally, it does not cause significant mortality but does require aggres-sive symptom management. Noninvasive measures such as oxygen therapy, fluid management, diuretics, and glucocorticoids may be utilized despite lack of evidence. Endovascular stenting has become the standard of care and unless contraindicated, should be incorporated into the initial treatment. The presence of rapidly progressing symptoms, evolving neurologic deficits or compromised

Table 3.2 Comparison of SVCS Treatments

Interventions	Advantages	Disadvantages
Endovascular stenting	• Rapid relief of symptoms • High response rates • Subsequent antitumor regimens may still be carried out • Well tolerated	• Invasive procedure • Does not treat underlying malignancy • Complications include SVC rupture, bleeding, stent migration
Radiotherapy	• Treats underlying malignancy	• Delayed onset of relief • Only certain malignancies are responsive • Treatment may be delayed until a tissue diagnosis is obtained • High recurrence rate • Complications include esophagitis, weight loss, skin irritation
Chemotherapy	• Treats underlying malignancy	• Delayed onset of relief • Only certain malignancies are responsive • Treatment may be delayed until a tissue diagnosis is obtained • Toxicity of individual anti-neoplastic drugs

ventilation warrants emergent stenting. Radiotherapy and chemotherapy may also be utilized, depending on the underlying malignancy.

Hypercalcemia of Malignancy

Approximately 20% of patients with cancer develop hypercalcemia of malignancy (HCM).[31] The incidence appears to be declining due to aggressive use of prophylactic bisphosphonates, particularly in breast cancer and multiple myeloma.[31] The malignancies most commonly associated with HCM are breast, squamous cell (often lung), lymphoma, and multiple myeloma. Up to 20% of cases occur without bony metastases. Approximately 50% of patients with HCM die within 30 days.[31]

Signs and Symptoms

Hypercalcemia of malignancy causes a spectrum of symptomatology. Mild cases (serum calcium levels of 10–12 mg/dl) present with nonspecific musculoskeletal pain and gastrointestinal complaints, such as constipation, nausea, and anorexia. These patients also may exhibit neuropsychiatric symptoms, such as anxiety, fatigue, and depression. As the serum calcium level rises, symptoms become more severe and include polyuria, polydipsia, and weakness. The severity of symptoms appears to correlate with the rate of rise in serum calcium, not simply the level of serum calcium. Moderate hypercalcemia, serum levels between

12 and 14 mg/dl, may be well-tolerated chronically but may cause delirium acutely. Severe hypercalcemia, a serum level > 14 mg/dl, tends to cause more distressing symptoms and often results in alterations in sensorium that range from confusion to coma.

Severe symptoms are more commonly seen in the elderly, who are more sensitive to fluctuations and disturbances in fluids and electrolytes. Children, on the other hand, appear to tolerate a relative hypercalcemia with fewer symptoms at higher levels. Pediatric HCM is fortunately only experienced by approximately 0.4%–0.7% of pediatric oncology patients.[32]

Pathophysiology

Hypercalcemia of malignancy occurs primarily via three mechanisms: (1) increased osteoclastic activity and bone resorption; (2) decreased renal calcium clearance due to decreased glomerular filtration and increased tubular reabsorption; and (3) increased intestinal calcium absorption. Therapies are aimed at targeting these mechanisms.

Interventions

Goals of care must be addressed, and patient and family expectations must be managed, in order to tailor therapy. Treatment of HCM is temporizing, and may improve quality of life by decreasing symptom burden. When possible, treatment may allow time for definitive therapy of the underlying malignancy. However, as prognosis is often poor, forgoing therapy might be a humane alternative in certain clinical scenarios. Untreated hypercalcemia leads to coma and ultimately death. Some patients and families may opt not to lower serum calcium, to allow natural death, and not prolong suffering through a protracted dying process.

When calcium control is the goal, initial management of HCM must include discontinuation of exogenous calcium supplementation. Secondarily, medications that increase serum calcium must be discontinued (e.g., lithium, vitamin D, thiazide diuretics).

Most patients with symptomatic hypercalcemia are profoundly hypovolemic from the decreased concentrating ability of the distal tubules of the kidney. Volume contraction often leads to acute renal insufficiency, worsened by decreased oral intake caused by nausea, anorexia, constipation, and increased renal fluid losses. Treatment of dehydration consists of fluid resuscitation with close monitoring of cardiovascular and renal status for volume overload. Once euvolemia is achieved, intravenous fluids are of limited utility. Historically, large volumes were infused with the goal of promoting calciuresis, usually in conjunction with loop diuretics, but current literature no longer supports this strategy.

Intravenous bisphosphonates are now the mainstay of therapy for malignant hypercalcemia. These agents are structural analogs of pyrophosphates, a naturally occurring component of bone crystal deposition. Their mechanism of action is multifold. They have a strong affinity to bone. They block osteoclastic resorption primarily by preventing osteoclastic maturation. Bisphosphonates require 48 hours to lower calcium and should be initiated at diagnosis. They must be given parenterally because oral absorption is very limited. Two bisphosphonates are currently approved by the FDA in the United States, pamidronate and zolendronate. The recommended typical dosing regimens are pamidronate, 60–90 mg intravenously over 2 hours, or zolendronate, 4 mg intravenously over 15 minutes. Pamidronate is less expensive, but zolendronate is easier to administer, more potent, and more efficacious.

A 2004 systematic review investigating the efficacy of bisphosphonates in the treatment of HCM, concluded that intravenous bisphosphonates are the preferred management.[33] Over 70% of patients achieved normocalcemia in 2–6 days with all bisphosphonates. Side effects are minimal, with fever being the most common. A double-blinded study by Nussbaum et al showed increasing efficacy of pamidronate with increasing doses, comparing 30 mg, 60 mg, and 90 mg doses.[34] Major et al found zolendronate to be more effective than pamidronate. More patients became normocalcemic with zolendronate than pamidronate, and the duration of action was nearly doubled at 32 days versus 18 days.[35]

Several case reports of bisphosphonates in pediatric patients with HCM suggest a similar effect and safety profile as in adults.[32,36] Bisphosphonates are recommended in pediatric HCM, despite limited pediatric evidence.[36]

A 2009 Cochrane review on the utilization of bisphosphonates for pain relief from bony metastases estimates a number needed to treat (NNT) of six.[20] Severe adverse drug reactions requiring discontinuation of therapy were one in eleven. Maximal response was noted at 4 weeks, with a similar response at 12 weeks. Based on this data, the authors recommend bisphosphonates as adjunctive therapy for pain relief.

A 2008 narrative review of the use of furosemide in HCM, which was historically assumed to be standard of care, demonstrates that this practice is not evidence-based. It may instead be associated with significant harm, causing worsening overall fluid depletion and electrolyte imbalances. In short, recent literature no longer recommends the use of furosemide for the routine management of hypercalcemia.[37]

Calcitonin reduces serum calcium and is a useful adjunct to bisphosphonates in HCM. Calcitonin is secreted by parafollicular cells of the thyroid. It reduces serum calcium by interrupting osteoclastic maturation, thereby decreasing bone resorption, as well as by increasing renal calcium excretion. Onset of action is 4–6 hours and duration of action is 48 hours, after which time efficacy is diminished despite repeated dosing, suggesting the development of tachyphylaxis, possibly secondary to receptor down-regulation. Toxicity is minimal and consists most commonly of nausea. Normocalcemia is rare with calcitonin alone, but in combination with bisphosphonates, it is an effective and useful secondary therapy.

Glucocorticoids block absorption of dietary calcium due to overproduction of calcitriol. They have a limited role in the management of HCM from hematologic malignancies, particularly lymphoma, which occasionally produces calcitriol.

Table 3.3 summarizes dosing, time of onset and adverse effects of the first and second line treatment options.

In the rare clinical scenario when adequate fluid repletion is not possible due to renal insufficiency or cardiovascular compromise, dialysis may be considered using a calcium-free dialysate.

Table 3.3 Treatment of Hypercalcemia of Malignancy

Bisphosphonates	Dose/Route	Adverse Effects	Onset of Action	Duration of Action
First Line Agents				
Zolendronate	4 mg IV over 15 minutes	nephrotoxicity, myalgias, fever	24–72 hours	2–4 weeks
Pamidronate	60–90 mg IV over 2 hours	nephrotoxicity, myalgias, fever	24–72 hours	2–4 weeks
Second Line Agents				
Calcitonin	4–8 IU/kg SC q6–12 hours	Nausea, vomiting, flushing, unpleasant taste, tingling in hands and pain at SC site	4–6 hours	48 hours
Glucocorticoids	e.g., Prednisone 60 mg po daily × 10 days	Hyperglycemia, hypokalemia, immuno-suppression	2–5 days	Days to weeks

In summary, HCM is common and causes distressing symptoms for patients and families. Untreated, it leads to coma and death. Effective, well-tolerated, temporizing interventions are available, and should be initiated at diagnosis if aggressive interventions are consistent with goals of care. Intravenous fluids should be administered and normovolemia restored. Intravenous bisphosphonates given immediately are the current standard of care. Zolendronate is somewhat more effective than pamidronate, although pamidronate is also very effective and less expensive. Calcitonin may be used in the first 48 hours while awaiting the onset of action of bisphosphonates. Furosemide is no longer recommended in routine management of HCM.

Conclusion

Malignancies cause distressing symptoms that may require emergent interventions, even in the setting of poor prognosis. Maintaining a focus on timely and efficient treatment with an understanding of the goals of care allows the clinician to negotiate a skillful approach to emergency care while preserving the dignity of patients and their families. Metastatic Spinal Cord Compression, Superior Vena Cava Syndrome, and Hypercalcemia of Malignancy are particularly important. Each syndrome has evidence to guide assessment and treatment decisions in the emergency department to assure optimal management and care.

References

1. Loblaw DA, Emergency treatment of malignant extradural spinal cord compression: an evidence-based guideline. *J Clin Oncol.* 1998;16(4):1613–1624.
2. Patchell RA, Tibbs PA, Regine WF, et al. Direct decompressive surgical resection in the treatment of spinal cord compression caused by metastatic cancer: a randomised trial. *Lancet.* 2005;366(9486):643–648.

3. Loblaw DA, Lapierre NJ, Mackillop WJ. A population-based study of malignant spinal cord compression in Ontario. *Clin Oncol.* 2003;15(4):211–217.

4. Lewis DW. Incidence, presentation, and outcome of spinal cord disease in children with systemic cancer. *Pediatrics.* 1986;78(3):438–443.

5. Prasad D, Schiff D. Malignant spinal-cord compression. *Lancet Oncol.* 2005;6(1):15–24.

6. Helweg-Larsen S, Sorenson PS, Kreiner S. Prognostic factors in metastatic spinal cord compression: a prospective study using multivariate analysis of variables influencing survival and gait functioning in 153 patients. *Int J Radiat Oncol Biol Phys.* 2000;46(5):1163–1169.

7. Husband DJ. Malignant spinal cord compression: prospective study of delays in referral and treatment. *BMJ.* 1998;317(750):18–21.

8. Rades D, Huttenlocher S, Dunst J, et al. Matched pair analysis comparing surgery followed by radiotherapy and radiotherapy alone for metastatic spinal cord compression. *J Clin Oncol.* 2010;28(22):3597–3604.

9. Colletti PM, Siegel HJ, Woo MY, Young HY, Terk MR. The impact on treatment planning of MRI of the spine in patients suspected of vertebral metastases: an efficacy study. *Comput Med Imaging Graph.* 1996;20(3):159–162.

10. George R, Jeha J, Ramkumar G, Chacko AG, Leng M, Tharyan M. Interventions for the treatment of metastatic extradural spinal cord compression in adults. *Cochrane Database Syst Rev.* 2008;CD006716.

11. Graham PH, Capp A, Goozzee G, et al A pilot randomized comparison of dexamethasone 96mg vs 16mg per day for malignant spinal-cord compression treated by radiotherapy: TROG 01.05 Superdex study. *Clin Oncol.* 2006;18(1):70–76.

12. Sorensen S, Helweg-Larsen S, Mouridsen H, Hansen HH. Effect of high-dose dexamethasone in carcinomatous metastatic spinal cord compression treated with radiotherapy: a randomized trial. *Eur J Cancer.* 1994;30A(1):22–27.

13. Vecht CJ, Haaxma-Reiche H, van Putten W, et al. Initial bolus of conventional versus high-dose dexamethasone in metastatic spinal cord compression. *Neurology.* 1989;39(9):1255–1257.

14. Marranzano E, Bellavita R, Rossi R, et al. Short-course versus split-course radiotherapy in metastatic spinal cord compression: results of a phase III, randomized, multicenter trial. *J Clin Oncol.* 2005;23(15):3358–3365.

15. Rades D, Lange M, Veninga T, et al. Final results of a prospective study comparing the local control of short-course and long-course radiotherapy for metastatic spinal cord compression. *Int J Radiat Oncol Biol Phys.* 2011;79 (2):524–530.

16. Sze WM, Shelley M, Held I, Mason M. Palliation of metastatic bone pain: single fraction versus multifraction radiotherapy. *Cochrane Database of Systematic Reviews* 2002, Issue 1. Art. No.: CD004721. DOI: 10.1002/14651858.CD004721.

17. Young RF, Post EM, King GA. Treatment of spinal epidural metastases. Randomized prospective comparison of laminectomy and radiotherapy. *J Neurosurg.* 1980;53(6):741–748.

18. Klimo P, Thompson C, Kestle J. A meta-analysis of surgery versus conventional radiotherapy for the treatment of metastatic epidural disease. *Neuro Oncol.* 2005;7(1):64–76.

19. Chi JH, Gokaslan Z, McCormick P, et al. Selecting treatment for patients with malignant epidural spinal cord compression—does age matter?: results from a randomized clinical trial. *Spine.* 2009;34(5):431–435.

20. Wong R, Wiffen P. Bisphosphonates for the relief of pain secondary to bone metastases. *Cochrane Pain and Palliative Support Group.* October 7, 2009.

21. Cheng S. Superior vena cava syndrome: a contemporary review of a historic disease. *Cardiol Rev.* 2009;17(1):16–23.

22. Wan JF, Bezjak A. Superior vena cava syndrome. *Emerg Med Clin N Am.* 2009;27:243–255.

23. Rowell NP, Gleeson FV. Steroids, radiotherapy, chemotherapy and stents for superior vena caval obstruction in carcinoma of the bronchus: a systematic review. *Clin Oncol.* 2002;14: 338–351.

24. Uberoi R. Quality assurance guidelines for superior vena cava stenting in malignant disease. *Cardiovasc Intervent Radiol.* 2006;29:319–322.

25. Kvale PA, Selecky PA, Prakash U. Palliative care in lung cancer: ACCP evidence-based clinical practice guidelines (2nd ed.). *Chest.* 2007;132(suppl 3): 368S–403S.

26. Yu JB, Wilson LD, Detterbeck FC. Superior vena cava syndrome—A proposed classification system and algorithm for management. *J Thorac Oncol.* 2008;3(8):811–814.

27. Watkinson AF, Yeow TN, Fraser C. Endovascular stenting to treat obstruction of the superior vena cava. *BMJ.* 2008;336:1434–1437.

28. Schindler N, Vogelzang RL. Superior vena cava syndrome. Experience with endovascular stent and surgical therapy. *Surg Clin N Am.* 1999;79(3):683–694.

29. Lanciego C, Pangua C, Chacon JI, et al. Endovascular stenting as the first step in the overall management of malignant superior vena cava syndrome. *Am J Roentgenol.* 2009;193(2):549–558.

30. Courtheoux P, Alkofer B, Al Refa" M, Gervais R, Le Rochais JP, Icard P. Stent placement in superior vena cava syndrome. *Ann Thorac Surg.* 2003;75:158–161.

31. Stewart AF. Clinical practice. Hypercalcemia associated with cancer. *N Engl J Med.* 2005;352(4):373–379.

32. Kutluk MT. Childhood cancer and hypercalcemia: report of a case treated with pamidronate. *J Pediatr.* 1997;130(5):828–831.

33. Saunders Y, Ross JR, Broadley KE, Edmonds PM, Patel S. Steering Group. Systematic review of bisphosphonates for hypercalcemia of malignancy. *Pall Med.* 2004;18:418–431.

34. Nussbaum SR, Younger J, Vandepol CJ, et al. Single-dose intravenous therapy with pamidronate for the treatment of hypercalcemia of malignancy: comparison of 30-, 60-, 90-mg dosages. *Am J Med.* 1993;95:297–304.

35. Major P, Lortholary A, Hon J, et al. Zoledronic acid is superior to pamidronate in the treatment of hypercalcemia of malignancy: a pooled analysis of two randomized, controlled clinical trials. *J Clin Oncol.* 2001;19(2):558–567.

36. Lteif AN. Bisphosphonates for treatment of childhood hypercalcemia. *Pediatrics* 1998;102(4):990–993.

37. LeGrand SB, Leskuski D, Zama I. Narrative review: furosemide for hypercalcemia: an unproven yet common practice. *Ann Intern Med.* 2008;149(4):259–263.

Chapter 4

Malignant Pain

Jan M. Shoenberger, MD and Susan C. Stone, MD, MPH

The Cancer Pain Emergency

A cancer pain emergency refers to new or escalating pain of malignant origin. The intense suffering caused by cancer-related pain is often the primary reason for an emergency department (ED) visit. It is estimated that 33% to 64% of cancer survivors experience pain, yet up to 82% are inadequately treated.[1] Uncontrolled pain is correlated with poor outcomes including significant disability. Unlike chronic, nonmalignant pain, malignant pain is typically a result of disease progression. After pain treatment has been initiated, it is critical to evaluate whether there is progression of disease. Ruling out emergent acute processes such as bowel obstruction or spinal cord compression is time-sensitive. The patient should also be examined for all reversible causes of pain, such as bladder distention, constipation, and effusions. Reversibility will help gauge whether to titrate medications acutely or more chronically. While the workup for reversibility is sought, pain should be treated. Pharmacologic as well as nonpharmacologic management strategies should be employed during pain emergencies.

The Emergent Pain Assessment

Pain Scales

Pain assessment is characterized by quality/character, intensity, location, duration, and exacerbating factors. In general, the longer pain persists, the longer it will take to control. There may be a tendency to judge a patient's pain based on external appearance with a resultant underestimating of a patient's pain. In these circumstances, trust may erode between the healthcare team and the patient. To avoid this, formal pain scales should be used to assess pain to include numeric, categorical, and visual scales. Always remember to ask the patient what is a tolerable pain level to them and what their baseline level is on most days. Understanding if the pain is intermittent (such as with movement) or constant is important. For a given patient who lives with daily moderate-to-severe pain, their external appearance may be calm and may be misinterpreted as mild pain but on standardized scales their scores will be higher. Psychosocial and spiritual factors may also significantly impact the pain experience and the emergency clinician should reach for the support of the interdisciplinary ED team to explore contributing factors.

Classification

Being able to identify the type(s) of pain will be helpful when selecting the correct analgesic(s) and complementary therapies. For example, there may not be an identifiable stimulus and the description seems to be neuropathic in origin. There may be a complaint of shooting or burning pain unrelieved by opioids. The neurons are deregulated and firing and this pain may require alternate drugs discussed later in this chapter. Other patients may present with severe pain that is visceral in origin, such as pain due to bowel perforation. These patients require rapid opioid dose escalation and will likely ultimately require high doses that prompt the providers in the ED to feel concern and fear adverse outcomes. In order to treat pain, it is important to understand the different types of pain pathways:

1. Nociceptive: Two types of pain fall into this category: *Somatic* pain is related to direct invasion by the tumor with actual surrounding tissue damage. Somatic pain is typically more localized. *Visceral* pain related to malignancy occurs in conditions such as bowel obstruction and peritoneal carcinomatosis. Visceral pain is usually poorly localized.
2. Neuropathic: Neuropathic pain related to malignancy may occur in the absence of direct tissue invasion. It may be due to "misfiring" of neurons. Characterized by a burning sensation and allodynia, it is often resistant to opioids. Neuropathic pain may frequently occur as a result of treatment with cancer-directed therapies, including radiation and chemotherapeutics.
3. Mixed-type pain: cancer survivors often will suffer from mixed-type pain including a combination of nociceptive and neuropathic pain.

Opioid Naïve and Opioid Tolerant

Knowing whether a patient is opioid naïve or opioid tolerant is a key factor. Careful medication history of what the patient has been taking, not just what they have been prescribed is central. Patients who have been taking more than 60 mg of oral morphine equivalents for at least 7 days (30 mg oxycodone or 8 mg hydromorphone or an equianalgesic dose of another opioid) are considered to be opioid tolerant. Patients who have not are considered to be opioid naïve.[2] Patients who are opioid naïve will often require lower doses and are at more risk for opioid side effects of sedation and respiratory depression. Treating pain in patients with cancer who chronically take oral doses of opioids in the outpatient setting can be a challenge in the ED because the total dose required to control severe pain in the opioid-tolerant patient will be much higher and often makes healthcare providers feel uncomfortable because their routine use of opioids in their practice is usually at a much lower dose.

Pharmacologic Management

1. Choosing an Algorithm

The National Cancer Comprehensive Cancer Network (NCCN)[3] and the American Pain Society[4] have comprehensive algorithms for management of acute and chronic cancer pain of various intensities. For all levels of pain, clinicians should: (1) understand opioid dosing principles, (2) anticipate and treat analgesic side effects, (3) consider adding adjuvants specific to the pain, (4) provide psychosocial support and education to the patient and family, and (5) optimize nonpharmacologic interventions. When initiating therapy, the provider should concurrently attempt to determine the underlying pain mechanism and cause in order to select the optimal analgesic. The patient's pain intensity, any current analgesic therapy, age, and comorbidities (such as renal or liver disease) may contribute to the decision. All regimens that include opioids should include a bowel regimen.

2. Using Equianalgesic Dosing Tables

It is imperative that clinicians use an equianalgesic dosing table when dosing opioids (see Table 4.1). This can avoid under- and overdosing errors. Patients often have been taking all opioids prior to arrival to the ED and the clinician should ascertain which opioid and exact dose the patient was taking prior to arrival, in order to gauge the equivalent parenteral or oral dose of opioid. Use of an equianalgesic dosing table avoids both under- and iatrogenic overdosing/toxicity.

3. Calculating Initial Dose of an Opioid

Dosing should be calculated according to whether the patient is opioid naïve or opioid tolerant. In patients not previously exposed to opioids, morphine is generally considered the drug of choice to begin with unless the patient has had previous reactions. It is inexpensive, easy to titrate, and found in almost every ED setting. In the ED setting, hydromorphone has the advantage of offering the opioid-tolerant patient a theoretically better chance of achieving pain control simply because providers are more comfortable administering a single intravenous push of 1 or 2 milligrams of hydromorphone but are sometimes uncomfortable administering the equivalent morphine dosage of 7 to 15 milligrams. Table 4.2 provides a suggested algorithm.

4. Advanced Age, Renal Impairment, and Hepatic Impairment

Opioid dosing needs to be modified in the extremes of age as well as in patients with renal and hepatic insufficiency.[5] Opioids should be dosed according to the creatinine clearance (see Table 4.3). Elimination of morphine and the metabolites is mainly renal with about 10% undergoing biliary excretion. Because fentanyl has no major metabolites, it is a good option for patients with renal failure. Fentanyl can be given transdermally, sublingually, buccally, and intravenously. It has high lipid solubility. Liver dysfunction should not be gauged solely upon

Table 4.1 Equianalgesic Doses of Common Opioids[1]

Oral Dose	Drug	Parenteral Dose
30 mg	Morphine	10 mg
7.5 mg	Hydromorphone	1.5 mg
20	Oxycodone	NA
30	Hydrocodone	NA

[1] Levy MH. Pharmacologic treatment of cancer pain. *N Engl J Med.* 1996;335:1124–1132.

Table 4.2 Initial Dosing Algorithms

Opioid Naïve

.Morphine is the first-line drug used to control severe pain.

1. Starting Dose 2–5 mg IV morphine sulfate or its equivalent
2. Re-assess in 15 minutes (60 minutes if oral)
   - If pain unchange.d or higher → redose and ↑ by 50–100% per dose
   - Pain score decreased 4–6 ↑ repeat same dose
   - Pain 0–3 → continue at current effective dose

Opioid Tolerant

1. Starting Dose is 10–20% of the total opioid requirements in the previous 24 hours (around the clock/scheduled doses plus as-needed doses).
2. Re-assess in 15 minutes (60 minutes if oral)
   - If pain unchanged or higher → redose and → by 50–100% per dose
   - Pain score decreased 4–6 → repeat same dose
   - Pain 0–3 → continue at current effective dose

Table 4.3 Dose Reductions in Renal Failure[i]

Glomerular Filtration Rate (GFR) (mL/min)	Morphine	Hydromorphone Hydrocodone	Oxycodone	Fentanyl	Methadone
>50	100%	50–100%	100%	100%	100%
10–50	50–75%	50%	50%	75–100%	75–100%
<10	25–50%	25%	Do Not Use	50%	50%

[i] Aronoff GR. *Drug Prescribing in Renal Failure.* 4th ed. Philadelphia, PA: American College of Physicians; 1999.

liver function tests but should take into consideration hepatocyte function. For many patients with malignancy who have primary or secondary (metastatic) liver involvement, the liver function tests will be normal, yet the liver function may be impaired due to limited functioning hepatocytes. Clinicians should examine a cancer patient's prior imaging (computed tomography [CT] or positron emission tomography [PET]) to evaluate the amount of liver involvement. A good rule of thumb in liver dysfunction is that *opioids should be half the dose and twice the interval.*

Dosing for children younger than 6 months of age should be 50% of the dose that would normally be given to older children and adults.

5. Routes of Administration and Pharmacokinetics

Intravenous administration is usually best to achieve control of cancer pain that is new or escalating. Intravenously administered medication reaches maximal plasma concentrations (Cmax) more rapidly than other routes and thus the peak effect is reached more quickly (see Table 4.4).

After IV injection, peak effect is observed in 10–15 minutes. Morphine can be given intramuscularly (IM), intravenously (IV), subcutaneously (SQ), rectally, epidurally, intrathecally, or orally (PO). Onset of effect after an IM/SQ injection

Table 4.4 Time to Maximal Plasma Concentration (Cmax)[5]

Route	Time (minutes)
IV—Intravenous	15
SQ—Subcutaneous IM—Intramuscular	30
Oral	60

is seen in about 15–30 minutes and peak effect occurs in 45–90 minutes. The duration of action is 4 hours. Therefore, morphine will need to be readministered based on the Cmax during titration. For intravenous morphine this would mean repeating doses every 10–15 minutes if the pain is still severe. When no IV is available, subcutaneous administration may be particularly effective through a 25 g butterfly needle. Patient-controlled analgesia (PCA) can be used to initiate and titrate dosing. If available in the ED, it should be considered. This is easier for both the patient and nursing staff. Typically, PCA is used for those patients being admitted or those going home under home care or hospice. The PCA simply simulates administering a patient-directed dose and a basal rate. The basal rate provides a continuous infusion mimicking a long-acting opioid and a patient dose simulating short-acting opioids. The PCA has a lockout where the patient cannot receive a patient-directed dose. Typically, 10 minutes is used because it follows the Cmax. Some providers start with the patient-directed dose and set a basal rate after 24 hours of monitoring.

6. Pain Reassessment after Treatment

Reassessment of pain is the key to achieving control of severe pain and is one of the most common reasons adequate pain control is not achieved in the ED setting. This should be viewed as similar to the charting done when nitroglycerin is used for chest pain. In a busy ED, it is difficult for providers to reassess pain every 15 minutes. When using IV morphine for pain control, the peak effect will be seen in 15 minutes, so this is the ideal time to assess whether the initial intervention has been effective and whether redose is needed.

7. Opioid Side Effects and Toxicities

Sedation and Respiratory Depression

Sedation rather than respiratory depression is the first sign of opioid toxicity. Though often feared, respiratory depression is uncommon when opioids are properly dosed using an equianalgesic dosing table, and carefully considering age, as well as renal and hepatic metabolism. In the rare circumstance that aggressive pain treatment with opioids results in drowsiness and slow breathing, the aggressive use of naloxone is highly discouraged. Instead, it is preferable to stop administering opioids and wait for the medication to metabolize using verbal or gentle mechanical stimulation to arouse the patient. If naloxone is deemed necessary, use diluted naloxone in a stepwise fashion. Dilute 0.4 mg of naloxone in 10 mL of saline and give 1 mL of this diluted mixture IV every 5 minutes until partial reversal occurs. Aggressive treatment with naloxone may cause a traumatic return of agonizing pain.

Nausea and Vomiting

Opioids may induce nausea and vomiting that will typically attenuate over the first several days of administration. It is not necessary to administer antiemetics routinely with opioids unless the patient complains of nausea/vomiting. For acute management, antiemetics are recommended. There is also the option of switching to another opioid given the incomplete cross-tolerance of opioids. There are many antiemetics to choose from and no one antiemetic has been found to be superior in this setting.

Myoclonus

If myoclonus develops, this is a known neuroexcitatory effect of opioids due to metabolites and is more common when the patient has renal dysfunction due to poor metabolite excretion. There are several approaches, including observation, if this is acceptable to the patient. Dose reduction by 50% is another option. Ultimately, rotating to a different opioid may work. Fentanyl and methadone (under the correct supervision) are good options due to lack of metabolites.

Constipation

All opioids cause constipation and patients must be started on a stimulant-laxative bowel regimen (such as senna, bisacodyl, sorbitol, or lactulose) upon initiation of opioid therapies. Failure to initiate a bowel regimen prophylactically can lead to constipation that results in anorexia, nausea/vomiting, obstipation, and/or functional bowel obstruction.

Confrontation of Barriers

Providers' fears of addiction, respiratory depression, and hypotension, for example, are often barriers to pain control in the ED for the opioid-tolerant patient. Education of providers is necessary to help them understand opioid safety as well as the definitions of addiction, pseudoaddiction, and tolerance.

Methadone

Methadone, metabolized in the liver, also has no active analgesic metabolites so no dose adjustment is needed in patients with severe hepatic dysfunction. Methadone, however, has limited use in the emergency setting and should be used under the guidance of a pain or palliative care subspecialist. The ED provider should understand how methadone is used in patients with cancer-related pain. Methadone acts as an N-methyl-D-aspartate (NMDA) receptor antagonist as well as a mu-opioid receptor agonist. This drug can be used to help prevent opioid tolerance as well as potentiate opioid effects, and is often efficacious in neuropathic pain syndromes. However, methadone has a very long half-life of up to 60 hours. This makes rapid titration unsafe. Reports of Torsades de Pointes and QT prolongation require electrocardiographic monitoring during dosage changes, which makes methadone a poor choice in the acute setting.

Nonopioid Pharmacological Management

Neuropathic Pain

Although opioids are the mainstay for the general management of pain in the patient with cancer-related pain, some types of pain may have a variable response to opioids and adjunctive therapies (coanalgesics) may be useful to achieve pain control. Neuropathic pain, for example, may or may not respond to opioid therapy. In neuropathic pain syndromes, other effective analgesics include tramadol, anticonvulsants (e.g., gabapentin and pregabalin). Additionally, antidepressants (specifically, tricyclics), corticosteroids, COX-2 inhibitors, and local anesthetics (e.g., topical lidocaine patch) may be useful.[6] If tricyclic antidepressants or an anticonvulsant are chosen, start with a low dose and increase the dose every 3–5 days.

Bone Pain

Bone pain from metastases may involve not only coanalgesics but also an interdisciplinary approach to management that may include radiation or nuclear therapies. Nonsteroidal anti-inflammatory drugs (NSAIDS) may be useful in the management of bone pain working as a coanalgesic, but must be used with caution given renal and gastrointestinal effects. Localized, focused radiation therapy or radiopharmaceuticals may be a very useful adjunct in controlling localized bone pain. When bone pain is diffuse, a trial of bisphosphonates or glucocorticoids (dexamethasone, prednisone) may be the solution.

Other Approaches

The emergency clinician should be aware of the many possibilities for malignant pain management that may not be achieved in the ED but nonetheless can be helpful to the patient. These approaches may be used for patients refractory to opioids and other adjuvant analgesics and will most often be administered by pain or palliative care subspecialists. In severe cases that cannot be controlled by typical management algorithms, other approaches may include low-dose ketamine or lidocaine delivered at subanesthetic dose. Interventional approaches include interventional nerve blocks, as well as epidurally or intrathecally delivered opioids and anesthetics. Other nonpharmacologic modalities may help control pain as well, such as heat and/or ice, massage, positioning, physical therapy, acupuncture or acupressure, transcutaneous electrical nerve stimulation (TENS), and ultrasonic therapy. Various cognitive-based therapies may also help control pain. Examples include hypnosis, meditation, imagery, distraction training, and coping therapies.

In summary, care providers in the ED setting care for patients with cancer-related pain on a frequent basis. Opioids are the mainstay of therapy to control pain, but many other modalities may be useful. Reassessment of pain in a busy ED is a challenge but is crucial in these patients because their pain can often be challenging to control.

References

1. Centers for Disease Control and Prevention (CDC). Cancer survivors—United States, 2007. *MMWR Morb Mortal Wkly Rep.* 2011;60(9):269–272.

2. Rappaport BA. Proposed transmucosal immediate release fentanyl (TIRF) risk evaluation and mitigation strategy (REMS). Website: https://www.tirfremsaccess.com/TirfUI/rems/home.action. January 4, 2012. Accessed August 12, 2012

3. National Comprehensive Cancer Network. NCCN Guidelines Version 1.2012—Adult Cancer Pain. PAIN-4 and PAIN-5.

4. American Pain Society. *Principles of Analgesic Use in the Treatment of Acute Pain and Cancer Pain.* 6th ed. Glenview, IL: American Pain Society; 2008.

5. Aronoff GR. *Drug Prescribing in Renal Failure.* 4th ed. Philadelphia, PA: American College of Physicians; 1999.

6. Levy MH. Pharmacologic treatment of cancer pain. *N Engl J Med.* 1996;335: 1124–1132.

Chapter 5

Non-malignant Pain

Jean Abbott, MD, MH

Introduction

Chronic pain is a common reason to seek care in the Emergency Department (ED). Painful conditions account for an estimated half to three-fourths of emergency department visits, with chronic pain accounting for 40% of those patients.[1,2] Emergency clinicians are caught between the duty to provide pain relief to their patients and the fear of contributing to the growing problem of opioid abuse, diversion, and death from overdose. Misunderstanding has led to frustration, variation in practice, and shunning of patients with chronic pain syndromes.[3,4] This chapter provides the principles to safely and effectively manage the patient with chronic nonmalignant pain.

Pain Pathophysiology

Pain is defined as "an unpleasant sensory and emotional experience associated with actual or potential tissue damage." It is a subjective experience, although it most often is initiated by noxious stimuli transmitted from the nervous system.[5] Nociceptive and neuropathic responses provide a structure to understand both the mechanisms and interventions of chronic pain.

Nociceptive pain "...arises from actual or threatened damage to non-neural tissue..."[5] Activation of nociceptive receptors is a normal part of a functioning somatosensory nervous system. The noxious stimulus is converted to an electrical signal from the peripheral nerve via multiple ascending pathways in the spinal cord to the brain. Nociceptive nerves are usually triggered by musculoskeletal damage, inflammation, or stretch or spasm of visceral tissues. The perception of pain improves as tissue healing occurs, usually in days to weeks.[6]

Neuropathic pain originates from a lesion or disease of the somatosensory nervous system itself.[5] Neuropathic pain results from abnormal function of the nervous system and is classically described by the patient as burning, tingling, shooting, stabbing, or electrical and may exist beyond observable injury. Etiologies can be central (e.g., stroke or phantom limb pain) or peripheral (e.g., postherpetic neuralgia or diabetic nerve damage).[5]

With persistent stimulation, nociceptive neurons may become overly responsive to normal stimuli and recruit adjacent nerve fibers. This is a process known as "sensitization."[5,6] Both central and peripheral damage from inflammatory mediators can sensitize nerve fibers so that previously subthreshold stimuli are perceived as pain, a phenomenon known as "allodynia." Structural reorganization of sensory neurons, ectopic excitability, and imbalance in sensory input occur as part of sensitization. All of these processes contribute to a transition from acute (adaptive) to chronic (nonadaptive) pain.[6] Opioids and other adjuvant medications work at different sites along the pain pathways. Timely medical interventions can blunt sensitization via inhibitory channels, while undertreatment and poorly controlled pain may encourage sensitization and exacerbate chronic pain.

Physiologic and Clinical Differences between Acute and Chronic Pain

Acute pain from nociceptive afferents interrupts normal patient activities and usually stimulates the sympathomimetic signs we associate with a patient in pain: restlessness, tachycardia, diaphoresis, and general distress.

Chronic or persistent pain commonly lasts beyond the expected time for normal tissue healing, which can be up to three to six months.[5] Chronic pain is complex in etiology and difficult to treat. While physicians are reluctant to rely solely on the patient's subjective assessment of the pain, this is the cornerstone of evaluation. The clinical picture of the patient with chronic pain can vary widely; several authors have described "pain justification behavior" in patients with chronic pain (i.e. exaggerated expressions of pain used to convince skeptical physicians that their chronic pain is real), even if they don't manifest acute pain signs and symptoms.[3] Various pain scales exist and are most useful not for a single measurement, but to serially monitor ED interventions and to establish the level of chronic pain at which the patient usually functions.[7,8] Vital signs, including respiratory rate, blood pressure, and pulse do not correlate with pain score.[9]

The functional consequences of chronic pain are wide-ranging, including physical, psychological, social, and even spiritual. Patients may become physically impaired and consciously limit activity in an attempt to avoid pain. Inactivity, depression, anxiety, and social isolation are common and may be counterproductive to maintaining and improving function. Long-term opioid use may further contribute to functional impairment by increasing pain sensitivity, depleting testosterone, and suppressing immune function.[10]

Definitions

The major pain and addiction medicine societies have developed the following consensus definitions[13]:

Tolerance:…a state of adaptation in which exposure to a drug induces changes that result in a diminution of one or more of the drug's effects over time.

Physical Dependence:…a state of adaptation that is manifested by a drug-class-specific withdrawal syndrome that can be produced by abrupt cessation, rapid dose reduction, decreasing blood level of the drug, and/or administration of an antagonist.

Table 5.1 Behaviors Characteristic of Addiction and Pseudo-addiction[3,12,13]

Addiction	Pseudo-addiction
Personal or family history of drug or alcohol abuse	Arguments over medications and dosing
Legal problems related to alcohol or drug abuse	Clock-watching
Losing prescriptions	Pain-seeking behavior that resolves when pain adequately managed
"Allergic" to multiple specific medications	Ability to consider a variety of options for managing their pain (e.g., nerve block)
Increasingly frequent visits if opioids prescribed	Openness to differentiating unacceptable side effects from true allergy to specific medications
Inability to control drug use, compulsive use, and evidence of craving.	
Use "despite harm"—to social situation, family, work environment	

Addiction:...a primary, chronic, neurobiological disease, with genetic, psychosocial, and environmental factors influencing its development and manifestations. It is characterized by behaviors that include one or more of the following: impaired control over drug use, compulsive use, continued use despite harm, and craving.

Pseudoaddiction:...drug-seeking behaviors that suggest addiction but instead are the result of undertreated pain and resolve when adequate pain relief is obtained.

Differentiating addiction from pseudoaddiction is particularly difficult in the ED setting. Many behaviors, such as amplification of visible symptoms to convince doctors of the "reality" of pain, doctor-shopping, and begging for more pain medicine, are seen with both, and addiction is the less common of the two, despite the provider's concern about not contributing to addiction. Table 5.1 lists some of the differentiating features.

General Principles for Managing Chronic Pain

Only rarely does the emergency clinician initiate a new treatment plan for chronic pain in the ED. Nonetheless, emergency clinicians need to be aware of some of the important characteristics of modalities and principles for chronic pain management:

- Opioids should be titrated for acute pain relief, recognizing the 6–10 minute time to peak pain control for intravenous administration, and the varied half-life of opioid agents.
- For chronic pain, opioids may not be effective. Improved functional outcomes are the most important measures of efficacy, requiring comprehensive longitudinal monitoring.

- Other common adjuvant pharmacologic agents for chronic pain include: anti-convulsants, antidepressants, corticosteroids, local anesthetics, and NMDA-receptor antagonists.
- Neuropathic pain, a major source of chronic pain, likewise is often poorly treated with opioids, which are considered second-line agents most useful for cancer pain or for acute exacerbations. More commonly, calcium channel blockers, alpha 2-delta ligands (gabapentin, pregabalin), and cyclic antidepressants or serotonin norepinephrine reuptake inhibitors (SNRIs)—more than selective serotonin reuptake inhibitors (SSRIs)—are used for neuropathic pain.[5]
- Patient-controlled analgesia is an excellent mode of delivery of steady levels of opioid analgesics, particularly in the patient on chronic opioids where there is a need to establish new opioid requirements.
- Many patients on a comprehensive chronic pain program will be on long-acting opioids that avoid multiple highs and lows during the day, plus short-acting breakthrough narcotics.
- Patients in pain management programs also may participate in a "contract" or "informed consent" agreement that spells out clinician responsibilities and commits them to obtaining prescriptions from only one source, to not ask for early refills, and to other treatment and behavioral modalities.[11]
- Regional block or low-dose ketamine can be useful if the patient is high-risk for addiction.

Policies Informing Emergency Department Management of Chronic Pain

The American College of Emergency Physicians (ACEP), in a position statement from 2010 has stated that "Management of pain is an essential nursing and physician responsibility....All patients should be treated appropriately for reports of pain, including those with addictive disease."[14] That same policy affirms that "aberrant behaviors do not equate with addictive disease and may indicate under-treatment of pain." ACEP has just developed a clinical guideline regarding critical issues for Emergency Medicine (EM) physicians in prescribing opioids to adults in the ED. This policy, which was finalized in 2012, provides an extensive review of the epidemiology of the growing problem of opioid diversion, risk factors for opioid abuse, and current evidence of the efficacy of various treatment modalities in acute and chronic pain. The policy recommends that opioids be used on a case-by-case basis for patients with chronic noncancer pain; that emergency clinicians honor existing physician patient-agreements; and that they only prescribe short courses of opioids if writing prescriptions following an ED visit. The policy recognizes the dearth of research regarding the best way to manage acute and acute-on-chronic pain, and emphasizes the need for careful history and physical, assessment of functional outcomes, and recognition of patient variability in needs and responses to opioids.[15]

Two Clinical Practice Guidelines from a coalition of pain specialist organizations (with EM representation) recently published extensive reviews and recommendations for opioid use in chronic noncancer pain, and for predicting aberrant behavior in patients on long-term opioids. The guidelines encourage comprehensive treatment programs for chronic pain, careful patient selection, close monitoring and a multidimensional therapeutic approach.[11] The panel also reviewed the limited evidence to date of effective tools for predicting and identifying aberrant drug-related behavior.[16,17]

An Emergency Department Approach to Chronic Pain

The overall goals of chronic pain management are complex and require longitudinal management or evaluation of outcomes such as the following:

- Reduce pain and decrease or eliminate opioid requirements
- Increase activity and return to school or employment
- Decrease health care utilization, including nonbeneficial surgeries and repeated exposure to imaging.[18]

In the ED, the goal should be to acutely relieve disabling pain, to reinforce and encourage good comprehensive care, and to discourage repeated temporary interventions that may be inconsistent with a reasonable plan. The general approach to the chronic pain is outlined in Table 5.2 and includes four overall steps:

1. Assess (history and physical examination)

It can be tempting to abbreviate the assessment for a patient with "chronic pain," but detecting a new deficit, recognizing pseudoaddiction, and understanding historical barriers to this patient's good management come from the history and physical. Careful assessment allows the provider to consider and

Table 5.2 Management of the Chronic Pain Patient in the ED	
Assess (history and physical)	• Careful history and physical • Search for new deficits, problems • Elicit psychosocial cofactors • Current and past medications (prn and scheduled), dosing, and most recent actual doses
Validate chronic pain history	• Obtain history of prior interventions and diagnoses • Validate medical history from medical records and prior ED visits • Search prescription monitoring program, if available
Categorize acute need	• Functional level and recent changes • New deficits that might require imaging • Identify reason for acute presentation to ED
Educate/document	• Document careful examination for future reference. • Document agreements with patient regarding follow-up and expectations for future ED visits • Communicate assessment/interventions with patient's doctor

evaluate for alternative sources of acute pain unrelated to the chronic problem, and to determine the need for emergency imaging or intervention. Because nonpharmacologic modalities such as counseling, physical therapy, and activity programs are at least as important as pharmacological interventions in managing chronic pain properly, these should be assessed and reinforced.

2. Validate chronic pain history

Given the concerns about opioid diversion and fostering nonbeneficial treatments of patients with chronic pain, the emergency clinician needs to make an effort to confirm the patient's verbal history. Although physicians worry about "being had," physicians often discover, during the validation process, that the patient actually has chronically undertreated pain.[2] State-based prescription monitoring programs have been shown to change management and prescribing habits in the ED (either prescribing less OR more opioids than originally planned), and hold potential for reducing opioid abuse, diversion, and overdose.[15,19,20]

3. Categorize acute need

Management of the patient with chronic pain depends on the reason the patient is presenting to the ED. It is helpful to categorize patients to direct the best management:

- Acute exacerbation of chronic pain (e.g., back pain)
- Unrelated acute painful complaint or intercurrent illness
- Acute painful flare of a chronically painful condition
- Stable chronic complaints with lack of access to ongoing medical care
- Aberrant drug-related behavior concerning for addiction or diversion

The physician should ask the patient to describe his or her expectations for the ED visit. These may be more modest than anticipated. A question such as "At what level of pain do you usually function normally?" can be useful. An acute flare of a known chronic painful condition, such as a sickle cell pain crisis, should be appropriately treated with aggressive acute opioid administration in the ED to break the cycle of pain and immobility. For the patient with chronic pain and an unrelated nonpain ED presentation, maintaining medications and preventing withdrawal is the most important consideration. Patients may require higher doses of opioids to manage acute pain, but even with a history of addiction, pain deserves our skilled management. The patient with acute nociceptive pain and a high risk for addiction may require opioids for reasonable pain intervention. Blocks; oral, intramuscular (IM), or rectal opioids; or subdissociative ketamine have been used if the clinician wishes to avoid intravenous (IV) administration of opioids.

Sickle cell disease (SSD) is the model of a disease in which there are acute painful flares of a chronically painful condition. Frequent presentations for pain to the ED generate considerable frustration for the patient and the provider. Often this population requires high doses of narcotics and makes frequent use of healthcare services. There has been considerable effort to refute some of the common myths about patients with SSD. The rate of aberrant drug-seeking behavior in this population is no higher and is thought to be significantly lower than that in the general population. Although many patients with SSD live with considerable pain, in one recent population-based study, almost 30% of SSD patients have no disease-related ED visits or hospitalizations in a year.[21] Patients with more frequent visits have poorer quality of life, more severe illness based on hematocrit levels, transfusion requirements, and frequency of pain crises and pain scores).[22]

Developing guidelines for pain management of patients with SSD and others with known severe chronic pain conditions can be helpful in encouraging early aggressive pain management as well as in relieving the staff frustration with patients who legitimately use the ED frequently. In one study, a pain management protocol for patients with sickle cell disease was introduced to provide timely parenteral narcotics. Visits to the ED decreased (with a corresponding increase in admission rate), clinic visits increased, and total admissions decreased over the 4-year study period.[23]

The patient without access to primary care, or one who lacks a physician willing to manage chronic pain, is perhaps the most difficult for the emergency clinician. It is helpful to have a designated person (such as a social worker or psychiatric provider) meet with patients and distribute information sheets to teach them how to access appropriate care locally. It is also important to reinforce that ED care is not in the patient's interest, and that the best practices for addressing the complex problem of chronic pain require multidisciplinary work over time. The emergency clinician is obligated to both educate and break the cycle of poor treatment by discouraging repeated episodic visits to an ED.

Several management principles are important to remember in achieving pain control for the patient on chronic opioids. Failure to control acute pain can indicate one of several problems: too long between titration dosing, addiction, diversion, or psychic suffering by patient. Aggressive acute pain management actually makes relapse into addiction less likely than if pain is inadequately addressed.

In the patient with evidence of addiction (Table 5.1) and repeat visits to the ED, it is appropriate to discuss your concerns about addiction with the patient while avoiding contributing to the disorder. The disease of addiction requires specific and complex treatment, and is not well-served by prescriptions. This diagnosis and conversation should be documented and the patient should be instructed in how to access appropriate care for this very complex problem.

4. Educate and Document

Patient education should be a cornerstone of ED care of the patient with chronic pain. Taking the time to acknowledge and name the problem of "chronic pain" and to teach the patient can help the emergency clinician demonstrate empathy and make patient expectations more realistic.

Establishing a central database of communication within an ED, which is HIPAA compliant, respectful, and secure, and references pain agreements, knowledge about PCPs or prescription patterns, or physician advisements regarding what frequent utilizers and others should expect at future ED visits is helpful to recognize patients at high or low risk for opioid abuse and to provide consistent care. One study demonstrated that the vast majority of patients suspected of abuse who were told they would not receive further opioids from the ED did receive further prescriptions, either in the same ED or another.[24] Electronic medical record-based communications or "flags" have the potential to allow the message and management of patients with chronic pain to become more consistent.

Emergency department records should be sent to the provider who manages the patient longitudinally if that provider exists. Case management can be integral in the development of guidelines for management of repeated utilizers of the ED for chronic pain. Consistent policies and "scripts" for ED providers and staff can reinforce a consistent message about the ED's commitment to best practices in management of patients with chronic pain.

Conclusion

Confirming a patient's chronic pain diagnosis and needs can be challenging. Many myths and pitfalls exist in managing patients with chronic pain. Inadequate pain management is more common than addiction and most physicians will develop a philosophy of how to manage patients whose presentation and agenda are unclear. By striving to maintain or improve patient function through careful assessment, intervention, and continuity-of-care plans, the ED can continue to serve as a legitimate partner in the effort to alleviate pain.

References

1. Pletcher MJ, Kertesz SG, Kohn MA, Gonzales R. Trends in opioid prescribing by race/ethnicity for patients seeking care in US emergency departments. *JAMA*. 2008;299(1):70–78.

2. Todd KH, Cowan P, Kelly N, Homel P. Chronic or recurrent pain in the emergency department: national telephone survey of patient experience. *West J Emerg Med*. 2010;11(5):408–415.

3. Todd KH. Chronic pain and aberrant drug-related behavior in the emergency department. *J Law Med Ethics*. 2005;33(4):761–769.

4. Tamayo-Sarver JH, Dawson NV, Cydulka RK, Wigton RS, Baker DW. Variability in emergency physician decision making about prescribing opioid analgesics. *Ann Emerg Med*. 2004;43(4):483–493.

5. International Association for the Study of Pain. IASP Taxonomy. Accessed at http://www.iasp-pain.org/Content/NavigationMenu/GeneralResourceLinks/PainDefinitions/default.htm, and Definition of chronic pain. Accessed at: http://www.iasp-pain.org/AM/AMTemplate.cfm?Section=Home&CONTENTID=7594&TEMPLATE=/CM/ContentDisplay.cfm&SECTION=Home , January 28, 2012.

6. Mirchandani A, Saleeb M, Sinatra R. Acute and chronic mechanisms of pain. In: N Vadivelu, Urman RD, Hines RL, eds. *Essentials of Pain Management*. New York, NY: Springer Science; 2011:45–56.

7. Optimizing the treatment of pain in patients with acute presentations. Policy statement. *Ann Emerg Med*. 2010;56(1):77–79.

8. Marco CA, Nagel J, Klink E, Baehren D. Factors associated with self-reported pain scores among ED patients. *Am J Emerg Med*. 2012;30(2):331–337.

9. Marco CA, Plewa MC, Buderer N, Hymel G, Cooper J. Self-reported pain scores in the emergency department: lack of association with vital signs. *Acad Emerg Med*. 2006;13(9):974–979.

10. Ballantyne JC, Mao J. Opioid therapy for chronic pain. *N Engl J Med*. 2003;349(20):1943–1953.

11. Chou R, Fanciullo GJ, Fine PG, et al. Clinical guidelines for the use of chronic opioid therapy in chronic noncancer pain. *J Pain*. 2009;10(2):113–130.

12. Lusher J, Elander J, Bevan D, Telfer P, Burton B. Analgesic addiction and pseudo-addiction in painful chronic illness. *Clin J Pain*. 2006;22(3):316–324.

13. American Society for Addiction Medicine (ASAM). Definitions related to the use of opioids for the treatment of pain: Consensus Statement of the American Academy of Pain Medicine, the American Pain Society, and the Society of Addiction Medicine, 2001. http://www.asam.org/advocacy/find-a-policy-statement/view-policy-statement/public-policy-statements/2011/12/15/definitions-related-to-the-use-of-opioids-for-the-treatment-of-pain-consensus-statement. Accessed January 26, 2012.

14. American College of Emergency Physicians. Optimizing the treatment of pain in patients with acute presentations. *Ann Emerg Med*. 2010;56:77–79.

15. American College of Emergency Physicians. Clinical Policy: critical issues in the prescribing of opioids for adult patients in the emergency department. *Ann Emerg Med*. 2012;60:499–525.

16. Chou R, Fanciullo GJ, Fine PG, et al. Clinical guidelines for the use of chronic opioid therapy in chronic noncancer pain. *J Pain*. 2009;10(2):113–130.

17. Chou R, Fanciullo GJ, Fine PG, Miaskowski C, Passik SD, Portenoy RK. Opioids for chronic noncancer pain: prediction and identification of aberrant drug-related behaviors: a review of the evidence for an American Pain Society and American Academy of Pain Medicine clinical practice guideline. *J Pain*. 2009;10(2):131–146.

18. Fikremariam D, Serafini M. Multidisciplinary approach to pain management. In: N Vadivelu, Urman RD, Hines RL, eds. *Essentials of Pain Management*. New York, NY: Springer Science;2011:17–30.

19. Baehren DF, Marco CA, Droz DE, Sinha S, Callan EM, Akpunonu P. A statewide prescription monitoring program affects emergency department prescribing behaviors. *Ann Emerg Med*. 2010;56(1):19–23 e11–13.

20. Gugelmann HM, Perrone J. Can prescription drug monitoring programs help limit opioid abuse? *JAMA*. 2011;306(20):2258–2259.

21. Brousseau DC, Owens PL, Mosso AL, Panepinto JA, Steiner CA. Acute care utilization and rehospitalizations for sickle cell disease. *JAMA*. 2010;303(13):1288–1294.

22. Aisiku IP, Smith WR, McClish DK, et al. Comparisons of high versus low emergency department utilizers in sickle cell disease. *Ann Emerg Med*. 2009;53(5):587–593.

23. Givens M, Rutherford C, Joshi G, Delaney K. Impact of an emergency department pain management protocol on the pattern of visits by patients with sickle cell disease. *J Emerg Med*. 2007;32(3):239–243.

24. Zechnich AD, Hedges JR. Community-wide emergency department visits by patients suspected of drug-seeking behavior. *Acad Emerg Med*. 1996;3(4):312–317.

Chapter 6

Symptom Management

Kirsten G. Engel, MD

Introduction

Although pain is the most common symptom among patients presenting to the emergency department (ED), patients with serious illness frequently experience a range of other symptoms requiring ED intervention. Nonpain symptoms can cause significant suffering and morbidity, and in turn, effective treatment can have a meaningful impact on patients' quality of life.

This chapter will address several of the most common symptoms, including dyspnea; delirium; anxiety; fatigue and weakness; insomnia; fluid management and edema; nausea and vomiting; constipation; and diarrhea.

Dyspnea

Dyspnea is the sensation of feeling breathless or experiencing air hunger. It can be a frightening symptom for patients, and distressing for family members and caregivers. Although dyspnea is a common symptom and is reported by up to 70% of cancer patients in their final weeks of life, the patient's subjective experience may vary.[1,2] As providers caring for patients and their family members, it is important to realize that a patient's appearance and objective signs may not correspond to reported symptoms. Patients who appear comfortable with a normal respiratory rate and oxygen saturation may complain of dyspnea, while others with objective signs, including tachypnea and hypoxia, may deny feeling breathless. Understanding this feature of dyspnea is essential to providing care and support for patients and their families.

In some cases, it is possible to readily determine the underlying cause of a patient's dyspnea, which most commonly involves disease processes directly related to the respiratory tract (e.g., bronchospasm, hypoxemia, pleural effusion, pneumonia, pulmonary edema, pulmonary embolism, or thick secretions), systemic disorders (e.g., anemia, metabolic disorders), or psychosocial issues and anxiety. In other cases, the etiology of the patient's symptoms may remain unclear after an initial evaluation. While it is appropriate to manage or treat any identified causes or precipitants for a patient's dyspnea, it is also vital to provide the patient with symptomatic relief, even when the cause of their symptoms is poorly defined. This section addresses the traditional medical and pharmacologic approaches to the relief of dyspnea, as well as additional complementary strategies that should be considered when caring for a dyspneic patient.

Pharmacologic Approaches

Oxygen

A time-limited trial of oxygen may be helpful for acute dyspnea in advanced illness. While oxygen may alleviate dyspnea in hypoxic patients, hypoxemia is only present in a subset of those patients complaining of dyspnea. Furthermore, in a chronically hypoxic patient, oxygen may not alleviate the feeling of dyspnea adequately, and may create an increase in anxiety or agitation due to the application of devices on the patient's face, which can be perceived as more uncomfortable. In addition, pulse oximetry or blood gas measurements may be misleading gauges in the effort to alleviate dyspnea. The goal is to improve patient comfort, and it is clear that oxygen may provide a placebo effect in some patients who are not hypoxemic. In a recent randomized-controlled double-blinded study, Abernethy and colleagues evaluated the effect of palliative oxygen versus medical air (room air with ambient partial pressure of oxygen) administered by nasal cannula for patients who were not hypoxic.[3] Their findings demonstrated no difference in patients' ratings of breathlessness or quality of life over a 7-day period; however, both groups indicated an improvement in symptoms during the study, suggesting that patients may achieve some benefit from the sensation of air movement alone. The results of this study emphasize the importance of nonpharmacologic strategies (see Table 6.1) that may provide significant benefits to patients and reduce or obviate the need for supplemental oxygen.[4–6]

Opioids

It has been demonstrated that opioids can help to relieve feelings of breathlessness without causing any measurable changes in the patient's respiratory rate or arterial blood gas.[7–11] The proper dosing of opioids for dyspnea, which is typically only a fraction of pain-management doses, has been shown to alleviate the symptom while not causing respiratory depression. In addition, this approach to opioid use for dyspnea in a patient near the end of life may actually prolong life in a more comfortable condition rather than hasten death.[4,5] Dose, interval, route, and patient characteristics guide safe and effective management. In opioid naïve patients, initial dosing may be as low as one-tenth to one-third of severe pain dose calculations. In opioid tolerant patients, doses may need to be increased to approximately 25% above usual breakthrough pain doses to alleviate the additional symptom burden of dyspnea.

Anxiolytics

Symptoms of breathlessness are frightening and frequently precipitate feelings of anxiety and panic. Benzodiazepines are the mainstay for the management

Table 6.1 Nonpharmacologic Approaches to the Management of Dyspnea

Provide sensation of cool moving air (e.g., from a fan or open window)

Change patient's position to improve comfort and breathing (e.g., elevate head of bed)

Limit the number of people in the room and provide an unobstructed view of the door or window

Consider nocturnal non-invasive ventilation to reduce muscle fatigue of anxiety and, although lacking in evidence for independently alleviating dyspnea,[12,13] they can be used to complement other interventions in relieving a patient's dyspnea.[6,11] The management of anxiety is discussed in greater detail in the dedicated section below, titled "Anxiety."

Complementary and Nonpharmacologic Approaches

A variety of nonpharmacologic measures, such as making simple changes to the environment or a patient's position, may help to alleviate a patient's feelings of dyspnea. In particular, the sensation of cool air moving across a patient's face (e.g., from a fan) may relieve the sense of breathlessness. This phenomenon is likely due to stimulation to the V2 branch of the fifth cranial nerve, which has a central inhibitory effect on the sensation of breathlessness.[14] In patients with severe underlying respiratory disease, such as end-stage COPD, there is also evidence for a marginal benefit from nocturnal noninvasive ventilation, as a means of reducing muscle fatigue that contributes to dyspnea.[12,15] The nonpharmacologic approaches to dyspnea management are summarized in Table 6.1.

Delirium

Delirium has several core features, including (1) a disturbance of consciousness (diminished attention and altered awareness of the environment); (2) a change in cognition (including memory, language, and orientation); and (3) a rapid onset and fluctuating pattern (typically develops within hours to days and changes over the course of a day).[5,16] Delirium is extremely common among patients with advanced, terminal disease and can be present in up to 85% of these patients during the final weeks of life.[16,17] Delirium presents as hypoactive, hyperactive, and mixed subtypes. Hyperactive delirium is characterized by agitation and frequently involves hallucinations and delusions. By contrast, hypoactive delirium rarely involves such dramatic features and is characterized by confusion in the setting of sedation and lethargy. The mixed subtype involves elements of both hyperactive and hypoactive delirium, which often present in an alternating pattern. Although the features of hyperactive delirium are more familiar to most emergency clinicians, hypoactive delirium is actually much more common.[5,18] The evaluation of patients with suspected delirium can be aided and facilitated by a variety of existing diagnostic and rating scales. Three of the scales best-suited for the emergency setting are listed in Table 6.2.

Table 6.2 Tools for the Diagnosis and Assessment of Delirium		
Tools	**Brief Description**	**Key Features**
Delirium Rating Scale[25]	10-item rating scale	Designed to distinguish delirium from dementia, other disorders
Confusion Assessment Method[26]	4-criteria algorithm	Allows for rapid assessment
Memorial Delirium Assessment Scale[27]	10-item assessment tool	Ideal for repeated measurements

Table 6.3 Pharmacologic Approaches to the Management of Delirium

Medication	Dosing	Indication and Additional Information

First-line
  Haloperidol
Alternatives
  Olanzapine
  Lorazepam
	0.5–1.0 mg IV or 1–2 mg po
	2.5–5 mg po bid
	0.5–1 mg IV/po*
		First-line for management; may repeat with 1–2 mg q2hr prn (max of 20 mg in 24 hrs)
		Indicated for patients not responsive to Haldol
		Indicated for hyperactive/agitated patients

* It is important to recognize that anxiolytics can sometimes precipitate or worsen a patient's delirium. This is particularly a concern for elderly patients and those taking opioids.

Table 6.4 Complementary, Nonpharmacologic Approaches to the Management of Delirium

Expose the patient to familiar people, objects, and sounds as much as possible
Frequently reorient the patient with review of the date, time, and place
Provide support to the family and address their concerns and distress

Delirium has many different causes, and it is likely that in most cases the etiology of delirium in palliative care patients is multifactorial. Among the most common precipitants of delirium are medications (e.g., opioids, chemotherapy agents, steroids, anticholinergics, or antiemetics) and underlying disease processes (e.g., central nervous system (CNS) disease, metabolic derangements, infection, or hematologic abnormalities). Management of delirium includes addressing suspected precipitants, controlling the patient's symptoms with medication, and considering nonpharmacologic approaches that may further help to alleviate the patient's condition. These strategies are summarized in Tables 6.3 and 6.4.

Efforts to control the symptoms of delirium should be accompanied by the provision of support and education to family members. It can be very upsetting for loved ones to witness delirium, since it is characterized by marked changes in a patient's behaviour and interactions. Because the onset of delirium in terminally patients often heralds impending death, it is critically important that family members are provided with appropriate support and resources.

Anxiety

Anxiety is very common among the general population of ED patients, but can be a particularly intense experience for patients with advanced illness. Nearly all patients with life-threatening disease experience anxiety at some point during the course of their diagnosis and management. At the time of presentation to the ED, it is important to be aware of a patient's anxiety level and, in turn, to consider the variety of factors that may be precipitating or exacerbating the patient's anxiety.

The many potential causes of anxiety include situational factors (e.g., a recent diagnosis, anticipated intervention or imaging, and fear of death); symptom-related factors (e.g., pain, nausea, or dyspnea); and metabolic or drug-related causes (e.g., hypercalcemia, hypoglycemia, and medication side effects). It is also important to recognize that related or underlying psychiatric disorders that cause anxiety may be exacerbated by the patient's illness and its management. Anxiety is often linked with depression and, in some cases, it can be difficult to distinguish anxiety from delirium.

The management of anxiety should include efforts to address precipitating factors and processes, but also may involve consideration of medication, as well as nonpharmacologic methods. Benzodiazepines are the obvious first choice to manage anxiety pharmacologically. While they often are effective, providers should be aware that benzodiazepines can contribute to delirium in some patients (especially the elderly and those on opioids).[5] Nonpharmacologic approaches include relaxation techniques and guided imagery.

Fatigue and Weakness

Fatigue and generalized weakness are common symptoms among patients with advanced illness. These symptoms can dramatically impact a patient's life by limiting the ability to perform and enjoy daily activities. As a result, fatigue and weakness can cause significant frustration and distress for patients, as well as their family members. As providers, it important to recognize that some family members may believe that symptoms of fatigue or weakness are signs that a patient is "giving up" and, therefore, education is needed to help families understand the causes of fatigue and best approaches to management.[19]

Although the exact mechanisms that cause fatigue are not well understood, in most cases, it is believed that a number of different factors contribute to a patient's symptoms. These elements may include direct effects of the underlying condition (e.g., atrophy of muscle in the setting of cancer or heart failure) or other related conditions (e.g., anemia, infection, or metabolic derangements). It is important for patients and family members to understand that multiple factors underlie the symptoms that are experienced by the patient. Depending on the circumstances, management and treatment can include efforts to address reversible processes, as well as to incorporate several pharmacologic and nonpharmacologic approaches that are summarized in the tables below (see Table 6.5 and 6.6). Increasing evidence suggests that the management of fatigue and weakness involves a balance of the complementary benefits of rest and physical activity.[20,21]

Insomnia

Insomnia is defined by specific criteria, including (1) difficulty falling asleep (i.e., taking more than 30 minutes to fall asleep); or (2) difficulty staying asleep (i.e., asleep less than 85% of time while in bed); and (3) experiencing symptoms at least three times per week with a noted effect on patient's function in the daytime.[1,22] Among patients with advanced illness, it is most common for them to have trouble staying asleep, rather than initiating sleep.[1]

Table 6.5 Pharmacologic Approaches to the Management of Fatigue and Weakness

Drug	Dose	Benefit	Side Effects/Complications
Dexamethasone	2–20 mg qAM, daily	Increases energy and feelings of well-being	Effects may decrease after 4–6 weeks
Psychostimulants (methylphenidate, dextroamphetamine)	Methylphenidate 2.5–5 mg qAM and noon, titrate to effect (10–30 mg)	Increased energy and appetite	Tremulousness, tachycardia, insomnia, and anorexia

Table 6.6 Complementary, Nonpharmacologic Approaches to the Management of Fatigue and Weakness

Stimulate the Patient
- Encourage patient to spend time out of bed; obtain equipment that will facilitate this
- Focus on activities that are most important to patient and reduce other ones
- Provide sensory, intellectual, and interpersonal stimulation for patient

Review Medications—Stop medications that are no longer appropriate and may be making the fatigue worse (especially antihypertensives, cardiac medications, diuretics)

Hydration—Optimize fluid and electrolyte intake to enhance hydration (as long as it is consistent with goals of care and appropriate based on the degree of hypoalbuminemia)

Evaluation of a patient who complains of insomnia should begin with an assessment of their usual and current sleep patterns. It is important to understand what they experience when they have difficulty falling asleep or when they wake up during the night (e.g., physical symptoms such as pain, nausea, difficulty breathing, and/or psychological symptoms including anxiety, nightmares, or restlessness). Other important considerations during this assessment include medication effects (especially steroids and antiemetics); other substance use (caffeine or alcohol); and sleep-wake cycle reversal (due to napping during the day). This information will help guide the management of a patient's insomnia. Pharmacologic and nonpharmacologic approaches to the management of insomnia are summarized in Table 6.7 and 6.8.

Fluid Balance and Edema

It is common for patients with end-stage disease to develop fluid-balance issues and related edema, which may be both uncomfortable and upsetting to patients and their families. Hypoalbuminemia is one of the most common causes of this problem and can be due to poor nutritional status and/or underlying liver or kidney dysfunction. Decreased mobility in the setting of advanced illness, as well as previous surgery, direct tumor effects, and complications of cancer management are also important factors that may disrupt normal fluid balance

Table 6.7 Pharmacologic Approaches to the Management of Insomnia

Drug	Dose	Side Effects/Complications
Antihistamines	Diphenhydramine, 25–50 mg po qhs meclizine, 25–50 mg po qhs	Anticholinergic effects; may develop tolerance
Benzodiazepines Imidazopyridines	Lorazepam, 0.5–2 mg po qhs Zolpidem, 5–10 mg po qhs	Dementia and delirium may worsen Fewer adverse effects than benzodiazepines
Neuroleptics	*See Delirium Management*	Especially for patients with day-night reversal and/or delirium

Table 6.8 Complementary, Nonpharmacologic Approaches to the Management of Insomnia

Sleep schedule—Establish and maintain a regular sleep schedule; cognitive stimulation should be provided during the day and not during the night; avoid staying in bed when awake

Avoid substances that may affect sleep—Avoid caffeine (including analgesics with caffeine) and alcohol (may cause a paradoxical awakening several hours after falling asleep)

Control pain—Use long-acting medications to control pain during the night

Mind-body interventions—Consider relaxation techniques and imagery

and contribute to edema. The management of these problems is challenging and there are no definitive approaches to treatment. Although one might want to consider administering intravenous fluids or even exogenous albumin, these interventions can actually lead to worsening edema with extravasation of fluid and denatured albumin into the soft tissues. Table 6.9 includes some important principles and strategies that should be considered in managing patients with edema.

Nausea and Vomiting

Nausea and vomiting are exceedingly common symptoms among palliative care patients. These symptoms have a profound impact on daily life and can make basic activities unpleasant or even intolerable. For this reason, these symptoms frequently cause significant distress for patients and their family members. While emergency clinicians are generally comfortable managing nausea and vomiting, symptomatic relief for this complex patient population can be aided by an enhanced awareness of the mechanisms that contribute to these symptoms and an understanding of corresponding strategies for effective management.

Symptoms of nausea and vomiting can be related to causes in the gastrointestinal (GI) tract, as well as the central nervous system (CNS). The neurotransmitters serotonin, dopamine, acetylcholine, and histamine play important roles

Table 6.9 Management Considerations for Patients with Fluid Imbalance/Edema

Diet—Encourage patients to drink and eat as they usually do. Patients should drink some salt-containing fluids (soup, sport drinks, vegetable juices) and not simply free water (tap water, coffee, tea).

Compression—Consider support stockings or compression bandages to help facilitate lymphatic flow. Combining compression bandages with physical exercise can help to promote reabsorption of interstitial fluid.

Mucous membrane care—Care for mucous membranes (mouth, lips, eyes, nose, etc) to prevent the sense of dryness that hypoalbuminemia and intravascular hypovolemia may cause.

Skin care—Be aware that edematous skin is fragile and excellent skin care is needed, including frequent routine inspection, the use of skin emollients, and the avoidance of harsh conditions (extreme heat/sun or cold).

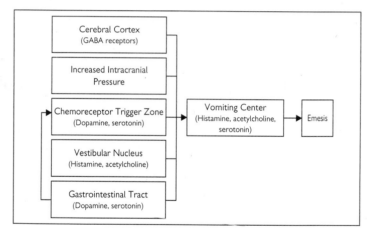

Figure 6.1 Pathophysiologic Pathways of Nausea and Vomiting

in triggering nausea and vomiting and the pathophysiologic pathways are summarized in Figure 6.1. Causes of nausea and vomiting that originate in the cerebral cortex are not associated with specific neurotransmitters. The cortex mediates learned responses, such as nausea, that develop in anticipation of chemotherapy and anxiety-related symptoms. This pathophysiologic framework makes it clear how understanding the etiology of a patient's nausea can help to establish which antiemetics are likely to be most effective in treating an individual's symptoms.[19,20,23]

While it is often not possible to determine the exact cause of nausea and vomiting, clinicians can usually identify a plausible mechanism to guide empiric therapy. Table 6.10 provides a summary of the major causes of nausea and vomiting, the underlying pathophysiology, and the corresponding effective approaches to pharmacologic management.

Table 6.10 Pathophysiologic Pathways of Nausea and Vomiting with Corresponding Management Strategies

Pathophysiology	Examples	Management
Cerebral cortex stimulation	Anxiety, learned responses	Anxiolytics
Gastrointestinal tract stimulation	Constipation, decreased motility, bowel obstruction, tumor burden	Bowel regimen, prokinetic agents Dopamine antagonists Serotonin antagonists Octreotide (to reduce intraluminal secretions in obstruction)
Chemoreceptor trigger zone stimulation	Medications (e.g., chemotherapy, opioids), metabolic changes (e.g., hypercalcemia)	Dopamine antagonists Serotonin antagonists Hydration
Increased intracranial pressure (ICP)	Metastases, meningeal irritation	Steroids, mannitol Dopamine antagonists Antihistamines
Vestibular stimulation	Movement-related symptoms	Antihistamines Anticholinergic

Constipation

Although it is a common cause for presentation to the ED, constipation is inconsistently defined by patients and clinicians. This variability can lead to problems with effective communication and management. Constipation is a clinical syndrome characterized by discomfort associated with a reduced frequency of bowel movements and involves a combination of hard stools, straining, and/or incomplete evacuation with two or fewer bowel movements per week.[5,20,24] While medication side effects (most common with opioids, but also with calcium-channel blocker and anticholinergic drugs) are frequent precipitants of constipation, there are other important causes including the patient's physical condition (e.g., poor oral intake/dehydration and decreased mobility) and the underlying disease process and its complications (e.g., mechanical obstruction due to tumor burden and spinal cord compression).

Preventive measures to avoid constipation should be considered by emergency clinicians, particularly in the setting of medication changes or increasing immobility or dehydration.[24] The combination of a stool softener and stimulant can be effective in ensuring that patients have regular, soft bowel movements even in the setting of limited oral intake.

The management of constipation needs to be aggressive because failure to address this problem can lead to complications, including pain, bloating, nausea, vomiting, overflow incontinence, fecal impaction, and bowel obstruction. Unfortunately, it is often not possible to modify the underlying condition or factors that are contributing to a patient's constipation, so management must

Table 6.11 Pharmacologic Approaches to the Management of Constipation

Mechanism	Etiologic Factors	Medication Class	Examples
Decreased GI motility	Medications, decreased physical activity	Stimulant laxatives	Senna Bisacodyl Prune juice Casanthranol
Stool with low water content, poor lubrication	Dehydration (poor oral intake, increased losses), slow-transit-time of stool	Prokinetic agent First-line: Stool softener Second-line: Osmotic laxatives	Metoclopramide Docusate Milk of Magnesia* Magnesium citrate* Lactulose Sorbitol
		Other considerations: Lubricant stimulants Large volume enemas	Mineral oil enemas Glycerin suppositories Water/soap suds

* Magnesium salts are contraindicated in patients with renal failure.

Table 6.12 Complementary, Nonpharmacologic Approaches to Management of Constipation

Increase fluid intake when possible.

Increase physical activity and amount of time seated, if possible.

Take advantage of the gastrocolic reflex (bowel movements precipitated by eating) and try to re-establish a pattern for having bowel movements that is consistent with patients' previously typical pattern.

focus on a combination of practical approaches and pharmacologic interventions, which are summarized in Tables 6.11 and 6.12.

Diarrhea

Diarrhea involves the passage of loose or abnormally liquid stools with an increased frequency. While acute diarrheal illnesses are most often due to infectious causes, chronic diarrhea is most commonly due to poor absorption, excessive secretions, or inflammatory causes. Medications can contribute to osmotic (poor absorption) diarrhea due to the presence of poorly absorbable solutes in the GI tract (e.g., magnesium-containing antacids or laxatives such as lactulose). Secretory diarrhea involves stimulation of increased secretions within the intestinal tract and is often caused by medications (e.g., laxatives, metformin, or diuretics). Inflammatory causes include infection, hypersensitivity, and chemotherapy-related causes that result in significant damage to the lining of the GI tract. Like other symptom management approaches, diarrhea management should first address any identified etiologies or precipitants. In addition, dietary changes (e.g., oral hydration solutions and gluten-free diet) can

Table 6.13 Pharmacologic Approaches to Management of Diarrhea

Loperamide, 2–4 mg po q 6 h, or higher;

Diphenoxylate/atropine, 2.5–5.0 mg po q 6 h or higher;

Tincture of opium, 0.7mL po q 4 h and titrated.

For persistent, severe secretory diarrhea:

Octreotide, 50 mcg SC q 8–12 h, then titrate up to 500 mcg q 8 h SC, or higher, or 10–80 mcg q 1 h by continuous SC, IV infusion.

often help to improve patients' symptoms and condition. Persistent diarrhea must be treated aggressively because it can lead to significant morbidity, including dehydration, fatigue, and perianal skin breakdown. Approaches to pharmacologic of diarrhea are summarized in the Table 6.13 below.

Summary

Patients with advanced illness experience a diverse array of nonpain symptoms that have a significant impact on their quality of life. The recognition and appropriate management of these symptoms are essential to caring for these patients. For the majority of these symptoms, it is important to try to identify and address any specific factors or precipitants that may be contributing to them. The patient's family and/or caregivers can be an excellent resource in the evaluation and management of these symptoms, and may benefit from education and emotional support. In all cases, the primary focus must be to relieve the patient's symptoms as quickly and effectively as possible. Both pharmacologic and nonpharmacologic interventions can be easily incorporated into the basic care of patients with advanced illness. Skillful management of symptoms can provide immediate and often lasting comfort to patients and families seeking relief of suffering in the ED.

References

1. Abrahm J. A Physician's Guide to Pain and Symptom Management in Cancer Patients, 2nd ed. Baltimore, MD: John Hopkins University Press; 2005.

2. Reuben DB, Mor V. Dyspnea in terminally ill cancer patients. Chest. 1986;89(2):234–236.

3. Abernethy AP, McDonald CF, Frith PA, et al. Effect of palliative oxygen versus room air in relief of breathlessness in patients with refractory dyspnoea: a double-blind, randomised controlled trial. Lancet. 2010;376(9743):784–793.

4. Kamal AH, Maguire JM, Wheeler JL, Currow DC, Abernethy AP. Dyspnea review for the palliative care professional: treatment goals and therapeutic options. J Palliat Med. 2012;15(1):106–114.

5. Bruera E HI, Ripamonti C, vonGunten C, eds. Textbook of Palliative Medicine. New York, NY: Oxford University Press; 2006.

6. Ben-Aharon I, Gafter-Gvili A, Paul M, Leibovici L, Stemmer SM. Interventions for alleviating cancer-related dyspnea: a systematic review. J. Clin. Oncol. 2008;26(14):2396–2404.

7. Allen S, Raut S, Woollard J, Vassallo M. Low dose diamorphine reduces breathlessness without causing a fall in oxygen saturation in elderly patients with end-stage idiopathic pulmonary fibrosis. *Palliat Med.* 2005;19(2):128–130.

8. Bruera E, Macmillan K, Pither J, MacDonald RN. Effects of morphine on the dyspnea of terminal cancer patients. *J Pain Symptom Manage.* 1990;5(6):341–344.

9. Johnson MJ, McDonagh TA, Harkness A, McKay SE, Dargie HJ. Morphine for the relief of breathlessness in patients with chronic heart failure—a pilot study. *Eur J Heart Fail.* 2002;4(6):753–756.

10. Mazzocato C, Buclin T, Rapin CH. The effects of morphine on dyspnea and ventilatory function in elderly patients with advanced cancer: a randomized double-blind controlled trial. *Ann Oncol.* 1999;10(12):1511–1514.

11. Johnson MJ AA, Currow DC. Gaps in the evidence of base of opioids for refractory breathlessness. A future work plan? *J. Pain Symptom Manage.* 2012;43(3):614–624.

12. Parshall MB, Schwartzstein RM, Adams L, et al. An official American Thoracic Society statement: update on the mechanisms, assessment, and management of dyspnea. *Am J Respir Crit Care Med.* 2012;185(4):435–452.

13. Simon ST, Higginson IJ, Booth S, Harding R, Bausewein C. Benzodiazepines for the relief of breathlessness in advanced malignant and non-malignant diseases in adults. *Cochrane Database Syst Rev.* (1):CD007354.

14. Schwartzstein RM, Lahive K, Pope A, Weinberger SE, Weiss JW. Cold facial stimulation reduces breathlessness induced in normal subjects. *Am Rev Respir Dis.* 1987;136(1):58–61.

15. Casanova C, Celli BR, Tost L, et al. Long-term controlled trial of nocturnal nasal positive pressure ventilation in patients with severe COPD. *Chest.* 2000;118(6):1582–1590.

16. Breitbart W, Bruera E, Chochinov H, Lynch M. Neuropsychiatric syndromes and psychological symptoms in patients with advanced cancer. *J Pain Symptom Manage.* 1995;10(2):131–141.

17. Bruera E, Miller L, McCallion J, Macmillan K, Krefting L, Hanson J. Cognitive failure in patients with terminal cancer: a prospective study. *J Pain Symptom Manage.* 1992;7(4):192–195.

18. Ross CA, Peyser CE, Shapiro I, Folstein MF. Delirium: phenomenologic and etiologic subtypes. *Int Psychogeriatr.* 1991;3(2):135–147.

19. Ross DD, Alexander CS. Management of common symptoms in terminally ill patients: Part I. Fatigue, anorexia, cachexia, nausea and vomiting. *Am Fam Physician.* 2001;64(5):807–814.

20. Shoemaker LK, Estfan B, Induru R, Walsh TD. Symptom management: an important part of cancer care. *Cleve Clin J Med.* 2011;78(1):25–34.

21. Porock D, Kristjanson LJ, Tinnelly K, Duke T, Blight J. An exercise intervention for advanced cancer patients experiencing fatigue: a pilot study. *J Palliat Care.* 2000;16(3):30–36.

22. Savard J, Morin CM. Insomnia in the context of cancer: a review of a neglected problem. *J Clin Oncol.* 2001;19(3):895–908.

23. Glare P, Miller J, Nikolova T, Tickoo R. Treating nausea and vomiting in palliative care: a review. *Clin Interv Aging.* 2011;6:243–259.

24. Ross DD, Alexander CS. Management of common symptoms in terminally ill patients: Part II. Constipation, delirium and dyspnea. *Am Fam Physician.* 2001;64(6):1019–1026.

25. Trzepacz PT, Baker RW, Greenhouse J. A symptom rating scale for delirium. *Psychiatry Res.* 1988;23(1):89–97.

26. Inouye SK, van Dyck CH, Alessi CA, Balkin S, Siegal AP, Horwitz RI. Clarifying confusion: the confusion assessment method. A new method for detection of delirium. *Ann Intern Med.* 1990;113(12):941–948.

27. Breitbart W, Rosenfeld B, Roth A, Smith MJ, Cohen K, Passik S. The Memorial Delirium Assessment Scale. *J Pain Symptom Manage.* 1997;13(3):128–137.

Chapter 7

Spiritual Suffering and Bereavement

Ryan Paterson, MD and Jean Abbott, MD, MH

Introduction

The experience of illness, particularly terminal illness, stimulates important spiritual activities for many people. Individuals construct and reconstruct their narrative, and they may struggle to understand the meaning and purpose of their lives. For some patients, this is a very painful exercise because serious illnesses are often accompanied by a sense of isolation and a crisis in identity. There is an immense body of literature supporting the fact that spirituality and religion, both viewed from the patient's and from the clinician's perspective, are integral components of health and well-being and play an important role in how people approach illness and dying.[1,2]

The National Consensus Project for Quality Palliative Care (NCP) and the National Quality Forum determined spirituality to be an essential element of care that is important to the patient's health.[3] Multiple studies have found that the majority of patients wish that their providers would address their spiritual concerns.[4,5] Patients believe that asking about spiritual concerns furthers trust in clinicians and has an impact on medical treatment. They believe that conversations about spirituality can improve the clinician's ability to advise patients and to provide hope at the end of life.[3] This chapter will discuss the roles that the clinician and chaplain each take in caring for patients experiencing grief and suffering near the end of life and the techniques for rapidly assessing spiritual needs in the emergency setting.

Definitions

Spirituality is the aspect of human existence in which individuals seek to find and relate meaning and purpose to their life in this world—be it through nature, the cosmos, or a higher power or God figure.

Religion is a formal structure through which a person expresses spirituality within a community. A religious community is then organized around common beliefs, attitudes, practices, traditions, and relationships.

Suffering is, as Eric Cassel has said, "the state of severe distress associated with events that threaten the intactness of the person."[6] While physical pain can cause suffering, often the biological symptoms are modulated by more global threats to a person's identity and existence. Suffering can also occur without physical triggers, particularly as patients take stock of the relationships, purposes, and meaning of their lives.[6]

Grief is the normal cognitive, emotional, and behavioral response to a loss and is often used to describe the broader, general response to loss.[7]

Bereavement is the state of experiencing a loss, usually of a significant person, through death.[8]

Pastoral Care is a specialized ministry that combines theology, psychology, and counseling. While chaplains are themselves members of a specific faith tradition, their expertise is in listening to patients and connecting the patient with the faith traditions and communities of the patient's preference. A chaplain is a vital part of the palliative care team who helps both religious and nonreligious patients address crises of faith that can be triggered by serious and life-limiting illness.

Grief: Normal and Complicated

Grief is a complex process by which a patient or family becomes reconciled to significant loss—of identity, of physical function, and ultimately of life itself. Although grief is commonly associated with personal or individual losses, grieving also occurs in response to larger tragedies, both natural and man-made. Classic stages of normal grief or bereavement were described first by Kubler-Ross in her landmark study from the 1960s. She described five stages of normal grief: denial-dissociation-isolation, anger, bargaining, depression, and acceptance. Various alternative models describing how people process loss, both emotionally and cognitively, have been described. The various stages are now recognized as an oversimplification of a complex process. Recent studies suggest that acceptance is actually the emotion most often experienced, even early following a loss. Disbelief, which may be exhibited particularly with sudden downturns witnessed in the emergency department (ED), is not universal or dominant in less acute situations. Yearning, depression, and other negative indicators often peak at about 6 months post-loss. The "work" of grieving can take up to 24 months to subside, yet grief in its entirety may never actually conclude.[9]

Adaptive grief is the progressive mixing of painful experiences of loss with positive memories and feelings that manifests over time as resilience.[7] The most important feature of adaptive grief is the attenuation of sadness and distress that allows increased capacity for engagement in life and the lives of others.[7] There is some evidence that patients with life-limiting illnesses accept their losses and adapt to their coming death better when they are aware of their prognosis.[10] Spirituality has also been found to be an important adaptive factor in grief and bereavement.[10] Several studies suggest that people who have spiritual or religious lives get comfort from their beliefs and have improved abilities to cope with such diverse threats as death of a child, pain, guilt, and fear.[10]

Complicated grief is the continued disability experienced by a minority of people when grief is prolonged and continues to interfere with health and the ability to re-engage with life. It is characterized by ongoing, severe separation distress and by dysfunctional thoughts, feelings, and behaviors that derail the normal evolution of grief.[7,11] According to proposals for the Diagnostic and Statistical Manual of Mental Disorders V (DSM V), the criteria set out for the diagnosis of complicated grief are: grief after at least six months from the loss with continued intense acute grief symptoms, such as the inability to accept the death, frequent thoughts or images of the deceased, a desire to keep objects of the deceased person near by, or to be with the person again, distressing thoughts/dysfunctional behavior, and recurrent intense rumination about the death that continue for at least 1 month. Such grief causes social, occupational, and life impairment and results in the inability to re-engage in life and the lives of others.[11]

Early mortality after bereavement is increased, and physical and mental health deteriorates for many people who grieve the loss of someone close to them. Increased use of medical services and psychological impairment, including increased risk of suicide, are reported. Somatization of grief may result in medical and ED presentations, and the variety of these expressions may vary across cultures. Risk factors for extended and complicated grief also have been suggested. These include loss of a child, traumatic or untimely death, multiple losses, economic threats due to the loss, low self-esteem, social isolation, and pre-bereavement depression.[8,12]

A "task" model of the work of grief has been described and includes a number of proposed projects: (1) accepting the reality of the lost person; (2) experiencing the pain of that loss; (3) adjusting to life without the significant person; and (4) "relocating" the lost person emotionally so that the grieving person can move on. It is important, however, to understand that coping methods vary widely, and denial or failure to discuss a loss is not necessarily a sign of a dysfunctional pattern. In addition, the length of normal grieving varies among cultures.[8]

Spiritual Needs in the Emergency Department

Role of the Clinician

Suffering may either masquerade as or be associated with physical symptoms, or it can be the explicit cause of an ED visit. The role of the emergency medicine (EM) clinician, as outlined in Table 7.1, is to recognize when the presence of existential suffering and grief are contributing to the patient's ED visit. In order to recognize this presence, clinicians must be unafraid to ask or respond to spiritual questions. The EM clinician also needs to be prepared if the patient or the family raise spiritual concerns. Even questions that seem, at first, to require an answer (e.g., "Why me?") instead require empathy, listening, and quiet curiosity from the clinician. The Joint Commission has recognized the importance of asking our patients about such matters and mandates that a spiritual assessment be taken of all patients.[13]

Most clinicians do not feel they have sufficient expertise to broach subjects of spirituality and religion with their patients.[14] In the United States, since the

Table 7.1 **Role of the EM Provider**	
Ask	Using spiritual assessment tool
Listen	To the patient's response
Recognize	The need for Pastoral Care
Refer	Call the Chaplain

mid 20th century, the teaching has been that it is unprofessional to discuss religion with patients.[14] However, most patients, even when not religious, now feel that it can be an appropriate discussion when pursued sensitively.[14] Curiosity about religious beliefs is, in reality, respectful and recognition has many important utilities.[15]

Recognition enables the creation of a medical care plan, referral to the chaplain for pastoral care, improved patient satisfaction and trust with their provider and it may attenuate suffering.[16] While clinicians commonly focus on "diseases," the patient's experience of that disease is the "illness." Understanding the patient's perspective, in its physical and spiritual dimensions, guides patient-centered care and avoids unwanted interventions. The role of the EM clinician is not to provide answers to a patient in spiritual crisis, but through the act of "respectful recognition," the clinician validates and honors the importance of this aspect of suffering.[14,5]

Role of the Chaplain

Once the patient's suffering is recognized, the clinician can then initiate a referral to a chaplain who's role is outlined in Table 7.2. The chaplain, as an integral player in the emergency care team, can help the patient explore these very difficult questions and journey with them as they come to their own answers. Certified chaplains provide a humane presence in the struggle for meaning as they journey with the patient.[17] Most chaplains will also be able to evaluate the patient's capacity to hope and other psychological struggles surrounding suffering. Using this ongoing assessment the chaplain can offer suggestions that may help the patient manage suffering, connect or reconnect the patient to the patient's community of faith, and offer encouragement during the process.

The chaplain is also very helpful in disclosing bad news when death occurs in the ED and in "being with" the family when the clinician is drawn back into the activities of the ED. While good studies are lacking, it is thought that family-witnessed resuscitation is at least not harmful to bereavement and may be helpful.[18] Viewing the body, and sometimes helping to clean the deceased

Table 7.2 **Role of the Chaplain**	
Humane Presence	Provide a companion on the journey of suffering
Tradition and Community	Help to connect or re-connect the patient to the patient's tradition and community of faith
Reflection on Spiritual Concerns	To be present and assist with reflection on religious and spiritual concerns
Disclosure of "Bad News"	Assist in the presentation of bad news in the emergency department

Adapted from *Education in Palliative and End-of-life Care* (EPEC); 2011, Module 14d[17]

person, may also facilitate the grieving process.[19] The chaplain can help to guide the patient's family members and to be present during these processes. Most important, the emergency care team may be the first to begin to help loved ones construct the narrative of this person's death—whether it is abrupt, or the expected end of life. Because bereavement is a process that usually lasts months, notification of the family's clinician is important for continuity of care.

Rapid Spiritual Assessment

The goals of spiritual care, as outlined by the specialty of palliative care, are to address the sense of isolation that accompanies serious illness and to work toward helping patients and loved ones find their own internal sense of meaning, purpose, comfort, strength, or balance.[17] While chaplains and the rest of the palliative care team will establish an ongoing conversation in the ED, a rapid method of discerning spiritual needs for patients near the end of life or for families beginning to grieve is also required. Taking a spiritual history is difficult and may be time consuming. It requires the full presence and attention of the provider.[10] The goal is to use open-ended questions that invite conversation, encourage spiritual questioning, and show respect for the patient's belief system.

While many approaches and tools exist to empower the clinician to take such a history, the FICA tool has been widely distributed and is readily applicable to emergency medicine. This tool provides a systematic approach to spiritual history-taking that allows patients to share as much of their spirituality or religion with the provider as they wish. It explores the patient's views on faith, the importance and influence of faith in the patient's life, and the role of community in the patient's life. It also seeks to determine the role of the medical team in addressing spiritual needs that are identified.

Table 7.3 outlines the four parts of the FICA Spiritual Assessment tool. Dr. Christina Puchalski designed this history-taking tool, which enables patients to talk about spiritual issues through a sequence of questions. The first set of questions is meant to explore whether the patient considers him or herself to be spiritual or religious. If the patient does not resonate with this, the inquiry can be directed toward a consideration of what are the patient's sources of meaning and purpose; this could include a variety of directions, such as becoming centered through nature or music or another transcendent reality. The second set of questions asks about the linkages between a patient's spiritual beliefs and the way they live their life, both in general and in relation to health and illness. Because isolation is often a part of serious illness, another set of assessment questions focuses on communities that might be a source of support for the patient. And the last part of the tool seeks to understand how the healthcare "world" should be linked with the patient's belief system and values.[16]

Common pitfalls in discussing spiritual and religious issues near the end of life have been outlined by Lo, et al. The clinician should resist the temptation to answer existential and unanswerable questions about the meaning of illness and why a patient is suffering. The clinician should not impose his or her own beliefs or attempt to practice pastoral counseling. Likewise, reassurance is not

Table 7.3 FICA—Spiritual Assessment Tool*

F—Faith, Belief, Meaning	Do you consider yourself spiritual or religious?
	Do you have spiritual beliefs that help you cope with stress?
	What gives your life meaning?
I—Importance and Influence	What importance does your faith or belief have in your life?
	On a scale of 0 (not important) to 5 (very important), how would you rate the importance of Faith/Belief in your life?
	Have your beliefs influenced you in how you handle stress?
	What role do your beliefs play in your healthcare decision making?
C—Community	Are you a part of a spiritual community?
	Is this of support to you and how?
	Is there a group of people you really love or who are important to you?
A—Address in Care	How would you like your healthcare provider to use this information about your spirituality as they care for you?

*Puchalski CM. Adapted from Borneman et al.

always possible; rather, the clinician should affirm the importance and difficulty of the spiritual questions asked by the patient.[20] Hope near the end of life takes on many forms, including desire to restore relationships, to not be a burden to loved ones, or to live to see an anniversary or special occasion. The clinician, as he or she explores spiritual dimensions, can sometimes help craft some realistic hopes for patients.[21]

Responding to Hopes for a Miracle

Patients and their caregivers experiencing serious illness may express their hope for a miracle. Clinicians may find such expressions an obstacle to discussing important end-of-life decisions, particularly in an emergent situation, and they may wrongly assume that such hopes for a miracle indicate a desire for life-sustaining therapies. Clinicians should be deliberate enough in their questioning to say—"Tell me what a miracle might look like to you." Regardless of the response, the clinician should (1) emphasize nonabandonment, (2) cite professional obligations to discuss the medical issues, (3) reframe meaning and manifestations of a miracle, and (4) suggest that a miracle can occur without clinician intervention.[22] Supporting the patient and their caregivers with clinical truths balanced with faith can enhance the patient-clinician relationship.

Conclusion

Clinicians traditionally have not been trained to delve into the spiritual lives of their patients. Patients, however, can suffer because of spiritual crisis near the end of life and often say that they want their clinicians to ask about their beliefs and the spiritual dimension of their lives. One contribution of the palliative care movement is to provide tools for asking. In the Emergency Department, it is important to recognize the potential for patients to present with significant suffering, with complicated grief, and in a crisis that goes beyond symptom management and biomedical interventions. The clinician cannot and should not provide answers for such suffering, but the emergency clinician is still an important link in the grieving process. By beginning the dialogue when this seems important, and affirming this part of being human, the emergency medicine team can connect people to pastoral specialists who can continue to explore healing and "wholeness" for patients near the end of their lives.

References

1. Post SG, Puchalski CM, Larson DB. Physicians and patient spirituality: professional boundaries, competency, and ethics. *Ann Intern Med.* 2000;132(7):578–583.

2. Koenig HG, Physician's role in addressing spiritual needs. *South Med J.* 2007;100(9).932–933.

3. Borneman T, Ferrell B, Puchalski CM. Evaluation of the FICA Tool for Spiritual Assessment. *J Pain Symptom Manage.* 2010;40(2):163–173.

4. Steinhauser KE, et al. Factors considered important at the end of life by patients, family, physicians, and other care providers. *JAMA.* 2000;284(19):2476–2482.

5. Sulmasy DP. Spiritual issues in the care of dying patients: "…it's okay between me and god". *JAMA.* 2006;296(11):1385–1392.

6. Cassel EJ. The nature of suffering and the goals of medicine. *N Engl J Med.* 1982; 306(11):639–645.

7. Zisook S, et al. Bereavement, complicated grief, and DSM, part 2: complicated grief. *J Clin Psychiatry.* 2010;71(8):1097–1098.

8. Stroebe M, Schut H, Stroebe W. Health outcomes of bereavement. *Lancet.* 2007;370(9603):1960–1973.

9. Glass RM. Is grief a disease? Sometimes. *JAMA.* 2005;293(21):2658–2660.

10. Puchalski CM, Dorff RE, Hendi IY. Spirituality, religion, and healing in palliative care. *Clin Geriatr Med.* 2004;20(4):689–714, vi–vii.

11. Shear MK, et al. Complicated grief and related bereavement issues for DSM-5. *Depress Anxiety.* 2011;28(2):103–117.

12. Maciejewski PK, et al. An empirical examination of the stage theory of grief. *JAMA.* 2007;297(7):716–723.

13. Hodge DR. A template for spiritual assessment: a review of the JCAHO requirements and guidelines for implementation. *Soc Work.* 2006;51(4):317–326.

14. Cohen CB, Wheeler SE, Scott DA. Walking a fine line. Physician inquiries into patients' religious and spiritual beliefs. *Hastings Cent Rep.* 2001;31(5):29–39.

15. Sulmasy DP. Distinguishing denial from authentic faith in miracles: a clinical-pastoral approach. *South Med J.* 2007;100(12):1268–1272.

16. Puchalski C, Romer AL. Taking a spiritual history allows physicians to understand patients more fully. *J Palliat Med.* 2000;3(1):129–137.

17. Emanuel LL, Bailey FA. *EPEC Trainer's Handbook.* EPEC, Chicago, IL; 2011.

18. Compton S, et al. Family-witnessed resuscitation: bereavement outcomes in an urban environment. *J Palliat Med.* 2011;14(6):715–721.

19. Williams AG, et al. Improving services to bereaved relatives in the emergency department: making healthcare more human. *Med J Aust.* 2000;173(9):480–483.

20. Lo B, et al. Discussing religious and spiritual issues at the end of life: a practical guide for physicians. *JAMA.* 2002;287(6):749–754.

21. Feudtner C. The breadth of hopes. *N Engl J Med.* 2009;361(24):2306–2307.

22. DeLisser H. "A Practical Approach to the Family that Expects a Miracle." *Chest.* 2009;135(6):1643–1647.

Chapter 8

Communication

Lynne M. Yancey, MD

Introduction

Communication skills are essential to the practice of emergency medicine, particularly when conveying life-changing news to patients and families. The information is often vividly remembered, and may have immediate and sustained effects well into the adjustment period.[1-4]

Effective communication in the emergency department (ED) presents a challenge for clinicians who have no prior relationship with the patient, are faced with persistent time demands, are confronted with complex and often unexpected events, and have incomplete data for decision-making. Emergency clinicians report having little training on the approach to difficult conversations, yet these communication skills can be taught successfully.[5-9] Using a structured protocol, for example, can decrease distress in clinicians delivering bad news.[10,11] In addition, nurses, social workers, chaplains, psychologists, or other professionals can provide a wide range of support to patients, families, and other hospital staff throughout these difficult experiences, and they should be involved as early as possible.

Breaking Bad News

Clinicians often discover disturbing information during the routine care of patients in the ED. Communicating this information can be daunting, even for the experienced clinician. Empirical studies and expert opinion offer successful strategies for these difficult communications.[12] Table 8.1 (SPIKES protocol) contains a simple, six-step approach that can be easily performed in the ED.[11,13]

S: SETTING UP the interview

The clinician should prepare for the encounter by reviewing any relevant medical information about the patient. It may also be helpful to mentally rehearse the conversation and prepare responses for likely questions from the patient or family. Arrange for as private a space as possible, and try to minimize potential interruptions by informing other ED staff that you will be delivering bad news. Begin the encounter by establishing a therapeutic connection with the patient or family—introductions, eye contact, sitting if possible, open and forward posture, and physical touch if appropriate.

Table 8.1 SPIKES Protocol for Delivering Bad News.*	
S—SETTING UP the Interview	Arrange for privacy
	Involve significant others
	Sit down
	Make connection with the patient
	Manage time constraints and interruptions
P—Assessing the Patient's PERCEPTION	Use open-ended questions
	Correct any misinformation
	Listen for denial or unrealistic expectations
I—Obtaining the Patient's INVITATION	Determine which people want information
	Determine how much information they want
K—Giving KNOWLEDGE and Information to the Patient	Warn listeners that bad news is coming
	Use nontechnical language
	Avoid excessive bluntness
	Give information in small chunks
E—Addressing the Patient's EMOTIONS with Empathic Responses	Observe for clues to the patient's emotional response
	Identify the emotion. If needed, clarify with open-ended questions
	Identify the reason for the emotion. Again, clarify if needed
	Allow a brief period for patient/family to express emotion
	Respond with an empathetic statement
S—STRATEGY and SUMMARY	Discuss next steps
	Verify understanding

* Adapted from Baile WF, Buckman R, et al. SPIKES—A six step protocol for delivering bad news: Application to the patient with cancer. *The Oncologist* 2000; 5: 302–311.

P: Assess the Patient's PERCEPTION

Find out what the patient already knows or understands about the situation. Use open-ended questions such as, "What have you been told about…?" or "Can you tell me what you already know about…..?" This step is allows the clinician to tailor the information to the level of the patient's current understanding.

I: INVITE the patient to hear information

Most people want to know accurate information about their diagnosis and prognosis. However, the level of detail desired may vary, as well as the patient's desire for family involvement in their decision-making. Possible approaches include questions such as the following: "I have your test results back. Would you like to discuss them in detail, or would you prefer a more general overview?" or "Would you prefer I discuss the results with you or with someone else?"

K: Give KNOWLEDGE and information

It may be helpful to "fire a warning shot"[14] such as, "Unfortunately the tests results are not good," or "I'm afraid I have some bad news." Proceed to discuss the information without using technical terms. Give the information in small chunks, followed by pauses to allow the patient to absorb the information.

If the results are not definitive, the preliminary nature of the results should be clear. Do not minimize the seriousness of the news—this may contribute to confusion and erode the patient's trust in the clinician. If the patient already understands the diagnosis, and there is enough information to accurately discuss prognosis, it may be appropriate to discuss it. It may also be appropriate to say that more information is needed in order to discuss how this will affect the person's future.[13]

E: Address EMOTIONS with EMPATHIC responses

Responding to emotional clues during conversation with a patient has been shown to be associated with shorter encounter times[9] and an increase in the amount of information gained during the same amount of time spent with a standardized patient.[15] Look for verbal and nonverbal clues to any emotion the patient may be experiencing in response to the news. Be prepared for a wide range of emotional responses, including denial, shock, anger, sadness, guilt, or even relief. Give the patient a short time to simply experience the feelings. Then acknowledge the emotion, and express empathy if possible. Examples include, "I can see this is painful for you. I wish I had better news," or "I know you weren't expecting this news. I was also hoping for a different result."

Offer support in whatever way possible. This may be as simple as offering tissues or a glass of water. It should also include reassurance that the clinician and ED staff will help the patient and family to deal with whatever immediate issues arise in the ED.

S: STRATEGY and SUMMARY

Finally, check in with the patient or family to assess their understanding of the information just provided. It might be helpful to have the person summarize what you have just said by asking, "I know this is a lot of information. Can you tell me what you understand about all this?" Clarify any misconceptions before moving on. Then negotiate mutually agreeable goals for further ED care, disposition, and follow-up.

Death Disclosure

One of the most extreme cases of delivering bad news is telling survivors that a loved one has died. This is particularly emotion-laden when the death has occurred unexpectedly, as is so often the case in the ED. Not only is it painful for survivors, but it is often stressful for clinicians. A structured approach to death disclosure can help reduce the traumatic impact of disclosure on both survivors and on ED staff.[16]

Advance preparation is one of the most important aspects of death notification. Arrange for a private space where family can gather. Have facial tissues and, if possible, a telephone available. Call for a social worker, chaplain, or other supportive healthcare professional to be present during the notification. This person is usually available to stay with family after the emergency clinician returns to clinical duties, and can be a valuable resource for the family and the ED staff. Make sure that the body is being prepared for the family to view, should they wish to do so later. Ensure that ED staff tending to the family

Table 8.2 The GRIEV_ING Mnemonic[1]

G—Gather; gather the family; ensure that all members are present.

R—Resources; call for support resources available to assist the family with their grief (i.e., chaplain services, ministers, family, and friends).

I—Identify; identify yourself, identify the deceased or injured patient by name, and identify the state of knowledge of the family relative to the events of the day.

E—Educate; briefly educate the family as to the events that have occurred in the emergency department, educate them about the current state of their loved one.

V—Verify; verify that their family member has died. Be clear! Use the words "dead" or "died."

___—Space; give the family personal space and time for an emotional moment; allow the family time to absorb the information.

I—Inquire; ask if there are any questions, and answer them all.

N—Nuts and bolts; inquire about organ donation, funeral services, and personal belongings. Offer the family the opportunity to view the body.

G—Give; give them your card and contact information. Offer to answer any questions that may arise later. Always return their call.

[1] Reprinted with permission from: Hobgood CD, Tamayo-Sarver JH, Hollar DW Jr., Sawning S. Griev_Ing: death notification skills and applications for fourth-year medical students. *Teach Learn Med.* 2009;21(3):207–219.

are clean and presentable, without bloodstained clothing. Review the patient's medical records, and be prepared to give as much accurate information about the events as possible. Lastly, make sure you know the patient's name and are comfortable pronouncing it aloud before you meet family members.

The Education in Palliative and End-of-Life Care—Emergency Medicine Curriculum[13] advocates use of the GRIEV_ING mnemonic[6] (Table 8.2) for emergency clinicians disclosing the death of a patient to the patient's family and friends. It has elements similar to the SPIKES protocol,[11] but is specifically geared toward death notification in the ED. This mnemonic was developed by and for emergency physicians, and has been found to improve the death notification skills of emergency medicine (EM) residents and medical students.[6,7]

Growing evidence supports that witnessing attempts at resuscitation may be beneficial to the grieving process of loved ones, without interfering with clinical care.[17,18] Communicating cardiopulmonary resuscitation (CPR) discontinuation, particularly in the presence of family, may be difficult for emergency clinicians. Table 8.3 describes a simple, structured approach recommended by the EPEC-EM curriculum that can be used with or without family present.

Special Considerations

Culture

A socially shared framework of understanding and interaction may be considered a definable "culture."[13] However, culture can vary widely within a nation or geographic region. In the United States, racial and ethnic minorities comprised over 36% of the total population during the most recent census.[19] Quest and Frank offer five evidence-based suggestions for emergency physicians to use in addressing cultural and spiritual diversity[20] (Box 8.1).

Table 8.3 A Six-Step Protocol for Discussing Stopping Cardiopulmonary Resuscitation.

Step	Example
1. Deliver a warning	"We have a six-year-old female who suffered a cardiac arrest secondary to drowning."
2. Recap events	"The resuscitation has been in progress for 105 minutes from prehospital to now with successful airway control, effective chest compressions, fluid resuscitation with two boluses of warmed saline, and correction of mild hypothermia from a core temperature of 34.6 to 37 degrees Celsius. Patient has been asystolic since arrival to the ED. Ultrasound shows no cardiac activity."
3. Allow the team to give suggestions	"Does anyone have any other suggestions for interventions that might help this patient?"
4. Explicit statement of team comfort about cessation	"Is everyone comfortable with stopping resuscitation?"
5. Pronounce death	"With team consensus, death is pronounced at 14:55."
6. Thank the team, acknowledge difficulty, and encourage processing	"Thank you, everyone. This was a very difficult case, and I appreciate everyone's efforts. Please take a minute to reflect in whatever way feels appropriate."

Box 8.1 Some recommendations for working with culturally, spiritually or religiously diverse patients[1]

1. Be cognizant and willing to assess divergent bioethical models of decision making
   a. Use open-ended questioning
   b. Involve the patient's family, caretakers or advisors
2. Use Translators whenever a language barrier exists
   a. Inquire with culturally concordant translators regarding word choice when applicable
   b. In order of preference:
      i. Hospital Translator: Same language and culture as patient
      ii. Hospital Translator: Same language
      iii. Hospital Translator: Phone
      iv. Ad-Hoc (not recommended)
3. Conduct a Brief Spiritual Assessment
   a. Particularly when high stress decision or end-of-life issues
   b. Be willing to call the hospital chaplain or the patient's own trusted clergy/advisors
4. Explore the Patient's Explanatory Model of Illness
   a. Use open-ended questioning to clarify how the patient defines the illness
   b. Check if the recommended care plan is acceptable within the patient's model
5. Respect and support cultural, spiritual or religious preferences to the extent possible in the emergency department.

[1] Adapted with permission from: Quest TE, Franks NM. Vulnerable populations: cultural and spiritual direction. *Emerg Med Clin North Am.* Aug 2006;24(3):687–702.

Requests to Withhold Information

Families may sometimes ask ED staff to withhold information from a patient about his or her own medical condition. Unless the patient has already indicated that she does not want to receive such information, it is unethical and illegal to withhold it.[13] However, rather than simply refusing to honor the family's request, it may be more productive to respond by seeking more information. Why does the family not want this information shared with the patient? Is there a specific fear or concern? Is there a particular cultural or religious perspective underlying the request? A possible next step would be to have a conversation with the patient and family together, asking the patient how much information she wishes to have about her condition.

Telephone Notification

Notifying family of a death or other bad news should happen in person whenever possible, but there may be times when the clinician must break bad news over the phone. Start by telling the person that they will need to be able to talk with you in a quiet place for several minutes without interruption. If the survivor is unwilling or unable to talk for several minutes, establish a specific time to call back, preferably within the hour.

When delivering bad news by phone, ask the family member to have someone in the room with them and to sit down, if possible. Clinicians can use the SPIKES or GRIEV_ING protocols to deliver bad news over the phone just as they would use them in person. Be sure to provide the survivor with the name and a telephone number for someone who can answer further specific questions about the event.

No Next of Kin Available

In some cases, a patient may have no legal next-of-kin, or it may be impossible to locate the next of kin. The Health Information Portability and Privacy Act (HIPAA) states that, for the purposes of notification, and when acting in a patient's best interest, one may assume that the individual has given permission to notify persons other than next of kin if no next of kin is available.[21]

Communicating with Children

Very little research is available on how to communicate bad news to young children. Usually a parent or guardian is present, and should be intimately involved in the process. If young children are present when a clinician is preparing to disclose bad news, particularly a death, it may be best to suggest that an adult take the children out of the room for a few minutes during the disclosure. The remaining adults may then experience their own emotions fully and privately. Then the clinical team can guide the adults on informing the children. Christ et al have recommended an approach to disclosing a death to children based on the child's age (see Table 8.4).[22]

If a child is the patient, and the bad news is a life-threatening diagnosis, start by informing the adults, and begin a discussion of how to inform the child. Existing literature indicates that children often become aware of their diagnosis and prognosis, even when not told directly. Keeping the information from the child often creates increased anxiety and a sense of mistrust, and may be counterproductive.[23]

Table 8.4 Recommended Guidelines for Families Following a Parent's Death

3-to-5-year-olds

1. Use concrete details to describe the fact that when a person dies, all bodily functions cease and the person does not come back.
2. Describe what the child can expect to happen next (particularly in the ED) and what role the child and other people will play.
3. Normalize emotions children and others might feel. Children this age may be frightened by intense expressions of emotion.
4. Offer the family any available resources for support groups or bereavement programs.

6-to-8-year-olds

1. Provide empathic support for initial responses to parent's death. Expressions of grief are often brief and episodic.
2. Children this age may ask blunt questions around the time of the death: "Are you a widow now?"
3. Reassure children that this is not their fault. Children blame themselves when bad things happen.
4. Offer the family any available resources for support groups or bereavement programs.

9-to-11-year-olds

1. If possible, give children honest, factual information about the diagnosis or events. Children this age often need concrete explanations to understand and feel a sense of control.
2. Normalize both emotional avoidance at this age and emotional outbursts sometimes followed by embarrassment.
3. Reassure children that this is not their fault. Children blame themselves when bad things happen.
4. Offer the family any available resources for support groups or bereavement programs.

Adapted from: Christ GH, Christ AE. Current approaches to helping children cope with a parent's terminal illness. *Cancer J Clin.* 2006; 56: 197-212.

Death of a Child

The death of an infant or child is one of the most traumatic events a parent can experience. It is also one of the most upsetting events for ED caregivers. After resuscitation attempts have ended and death has been declared, families should be offered the chance to stay with the child. They may wish to hold, rock, or bathe the child. This time is often identified by families as a defining point in the grieving process. Most parents choose to see their dead child and few regret this decision, even if the body is mutilated. In retrospect, parents often regret not being given the opportunity to see their child after death, even if it had been their choice at the time to not visualize the body.[24,25] Families place great importance on any personal effects or clothing; treat these items with care and respect and return them to the family as soon as possible. It may be particularly meaningful to provide a lock of hair, or a handprint or footprint (obtain ink pads from the newborn nursery).

Although the clinician must consider nonaccidental trauma as a cause for any unexplained pediatric death, it is important during the ED course not to suggest that a parent or caregiver is responsible. No matter what the circumstances, family should be offered the chance to be with the child and have some item of remembrance.

Sudden Infant Death Syndrome

Sudden Infant Death Syndrome (SIDS) is defined as the sudden death of an infant under one year of age, which remains unexplained after a thorough case investigation, including a complete autopsy, examination of the death scene, and review of the clinical history.[26] Approximately 80% of infants who suffer unexpected death will ultimately be found to have SIDS.[27] However, extensive investigation is required to establish the diagnosis of SIDS; by definition, it cannot be diagnosed in the Emergency Department. Clinicians should avoid making a premature diagnosis, and instead prepare family and caregivers for the investigation that will ensue.

Miscarriage or Stillbirth

Miscarriage and stillbirth are fairly common events in the ED. It is easy, particularly with early miscarriages, for healthcare providers to underestimate the potential impact of these events on expectant parents. Remember that while miscarriage is a frequent event in the emergency department, it is not a mundane experience for the patient and family. It is still a death and a loss, and should be treated as such. If possible, offer resources to the survivors, including any information about counseling and support groups that might be available. Offer to call a chaplain or other spiritual support person if the family so desires.

With the advent of bedside ultrasound in the emergency department, patients and family members are often watching an emergency physician perform the ultrasound, as well as watching the images as they appear on the monitor. It is common for anxious parents and families to ask about the results as the examination is being performed. It is best not to answer these concerns in a partial or vague manner. Unless a clinician is certain of the diagnosis and has the time to do a full death disclosure according to the model previously described, it may be preferable to say something like "I need to consider/review all the information before I give you an answer."[13]

Self-care and the Care of Other Emergency Department Staff

Delivering bad news and managing death in the ED is universally difficult for clinicians and staff. This is particularly true when the patient is known to the staff, if the patient is an infant or child, or if violence was involved. Often after such an event has occurred, the staff may feel pressured to immediately continue the work of caring for other patients. Although it may be logistically challenging to

Table 8.5 Communication Pearls

Make introductions in a respectful manner	• Introduce yourself by name, using formal titles (Mr./Ms./Dr.). • Shake hands if appropriate.
Be aware of nonverbal communication	• Make eye contact. • Sit down. • Remove any physical barriers between oneself and the patient. • Watch for nonverbal cues from others, such as frowning, avoiding eye contact, and crossing arms.
Begin with listening	• Use open directive questions and empathic statements. • Periodically summarize what the other person has said, and ask for feedback as to your accuracy.
Tailor the information to the situation and the person with whom you are communicating	• Find out what the other person already knows, and how much he or she wants to hear, in order to provide information that is most meaningful. • Avoid medical jargon.

call the staff together to debrief a stressful incident, it can be very helpful to all involved. Such a meeting need only take a few minutes, and can even happen at the bedside before the team disbands. A bedside debrief may offer care team members the opportunity to review events and express concerns or emotions that would otherwise distract them from their ongoing clinical care duties. In addition, they may draw support from their colleagues. Physicians are often in a position of leadership, where they may be able to call such a brief meeting more easily than other team members. More in-depth analysis of cases in the context of a "morbidity and mortality" conference may also provide a place for physicians and other staff to make sense of the events; share frustrations, sadness, or anger; and continue the work of healing so they can continue to care for patients.

Conflict

Sources of conflict around end-of-life care may include differences between clinicians and patients or family regarding goals of care, differing opinions among clinical-care team members regarding treatment or disposition, or differing opinions among family members regarding these same issues.

According to Patterson et al., conversations where conflict arises usually contain the following three elements:[28]

1. Opposing opinions: there are two or more opinions about the same situation.
2. Strong emotions: the issue is something those involved care deeply about.
3. High stakes: the outcome could have a huge impact on one or more of the persons involved.

A number of factors may contribute to patient or family perceptions of such a conversation:

- The degree to which the patient or family perceives there to be suffering, whether physical, psychological, or spiritual.
- Family structure and roles. These may be particularly important when a family member is functioning as a caregiver or medical decision-maker, or when roles change suddenly, as when a family patriarch is suddenly dependent on others for care.
- Stage in the life cycle. People are more accepting of illness and death in old age than in young adults or children.
- Family patterns of communication, whether healthy or unhealthy.
- Cultural or religious norms and values.
- Individual coping ability—both the patient's and the family's.
- Socioeconomic pressures, particularly financial resources or lack thereof.[13]

Conflict may manifest in obvious ways, such as verbal disagreements, or in confrontational behavior, such as demanding inappropriate or nonbeneficial interventions. More passively, patients or families may demand excessive time and attention, or refuse involvement during a time of crisis.

Staff may respond to these behaviors with counterproductive attitudes and behaviors of their own. They may take these behaviors personally and become defensive. Sometimes, patients or families are labeled "difficult," and staff may avoid contact with them. This can cause further anger or anxiety on the part of the patient or family, and contribute to an escalating pattern of negative feelings and behavior for all involved.

Stone and colleagues suggest a systematic five-step approach to difficult conversations.[28] These steps are summarized below:

1. Analyze your own implicit assumptions about the event and the parties involved.
2. Identify what needs to happen as a result of the conversation.
3. Find a neutral starting point, such as a shared priority, for beginning the conversation.
4. Seek to understand and acknowledge the other person's perceptions and feelings about the events.
5. Create solutions that meet both parties' most important needs and concerns.

Sometimes it is not possible to reach an agreement in the ED. If the conversation becomes stalled, ask for help. Bringing in an impartial outsider, such as a social worker, chaplain, or other mediator may allow a difficult conversation to move forward.

Summary

Many conversations in the Emergency Department are challenging. The most difficult involve high stakes, high emotions, and differing opinions. Having a standard approach to these conversations can make them easier and more effective. Table 8.5 summarizes some communication "pearls" that apply to any difficult conversation.

References

1. Mager WM, Andrykowski MA. Communication in the cancer 'bad news' consultation: patient perceptions and psychological adjustment. *Psychooncology.* 2002;11(1):35–46.

2. Sardell AN, Trierweiler SJ. Disclosing the cancer diagnosis. Procedures that influence patient hopefulness. *Cancer.* 1993;72(11):3355–3365.

3. Roberts CS, Cox CE, Reintgen DS, Baile WF, Gibertini M. Influence of physician communication on newly diagnosed breast patients' psychologic adjustment and decision-making. *Cancer.* 1994;74(suppl 1):336–341.

4. Butow PN, Kazemi JN, Beeney LJ, Griffin AM, Dunn SM, Tattersall MH. When the diagnosis is cancer: patient communication experiences and preferences. *Cancer.* 1996;77(12):2630–2637.

5. de Haes H, Teunissen S. Communication in palliative care: a review of recent literature. *Curr Opin Oncol.* 2005;17(4):345–350.

6. Hobgood C, Harward D, Newton K, Davis W. The educational intervention "GRIEV ING" improves the death notification skills of residents. *Acad Emerg Med.* 2005;12(4):296–301.

7. Hobgood CD, Tamayo-Sarver JH, Hollar DW Jr, Sawning S. Griev_Ing: death notification skills and applications for fourth-year medical students. *Teach Learn Med.* 2009;21(3):207–219.

8. Fallowfield L, Jenkins V, Farewell V, Solis-Trapala I. Enduring impact of communication skills training: results of a 12-month follow-up. *Br J Cancer.* 2003;89(8):1445–1449.

9. Levinson W, Gorawara-Bhat R, Lamb J. A study of patient clues and physician responses in primary care and surgical settings. *JAMA.* 2000;284(8):1021–1027.

10. Hammond I, Franche RL, Black DM, Gaudette S. The radiologist and the patient: breaking bad news. *Can Assoc Radiol J.* 1999;50(4):233–234.

11. Baile WF, Buckman R, Lenzi R, Glober G, Beale EA, Kudelka AP. SPIKES—A six-step protocol for delivering bad news: application to the patient with cancer. *Oncologist.* 2000;5(4):302–311.

12. Ptacek JT, Eberhardt TL. Breaking bad news. A review of the literature. *JAMA.* 1996;276(6):496–502.

13. Emanuel LL QT, ed. *The Education for Physicians on End-of-Life Care-Emergency Medicine (EPEC-EM) Curriculum.* The EPEC Project. Princeton, NJ: Robert Wood Johnson Foundation; 2008.

14. Barclay JS, Blackhall LJ, Tulsky JA. Communication strategies and cultural issues in the delivery of bad news. *J Palliat Med.* 2007;10(4):958–977.

15. Maguire P, Faulkner A, Booth K, Elliott C, Hillier V. Helping cancer patients disclose their concerns. *Eur J Cancer.* 1996;32A(1):78–81.

16. Adamowski K, Dickinson G, Weitzman B, Roessler C, Carter-Snell C. Sudden unexpected death in the emergency department: caring for the survivors. *CMAJ.* 1993;149(10):1445–1451.

17. Critchell CD, Marik PE. Should family members be present during cardiopulmonary resuscitation? A review of the literature. *Am J Hosp Palliat Care.* 2007;24(4):311–317.

18. Terzi AB, Aggelidou D. Witnessed resuscitation: beneficial or detrimental? *J Cardiovasc Nurs.* 2008;23(1):74–78.

19. Humes KR JN, Ramirez RR. Overview of Race and Hispanic Origin: 2010. 2011. Saunders, Philadelphia.

20. Quest TE, Franks NM. Vulnerable populations: cultural and spiritual direction. Emerg Med Clin North Am. 2006;24(3):687–702.

21. Privacy USDoHaHSOfCR, Rule Summary, 2013. http://www.hhs.gov/ocr/privacy/hipaa/understanding/summary/privacysummary.pdf. Accessed January 1.

22. Christ GH, Christ AE. Current approaches to helping children cope with a parent's terminal illness. CA Cancer J Clin. 2006;56(4):197–212.

23. Levetown M. Communicating with children and families: from everyday interactions to skill in conveying distressing information. Pediatrics. 2008;121(5):e1441–1460.

24. Finlay I, Dallimore D. Your child is dead. BMJ. 1991;302(6791):1524–1525.

25. Parrish GA, Holdren KS, Skiendzielewski JJ, Lumpkin OA. Emergency department experience with sudden death: a survey of survivors. Ann Emerg Med. 1987;16(7):792–796.

26. Willinger M, James LS, Catz C. Defining the sudden infant death syndrome (SIDS): deliberations of an expert panel convened by the National Institute of Child Health and Human Development. Pediatr Pathol. 1991;11(5):677–684.

27. Hunt CE. Sudden infant death syndrome and other causes of infant mortality: diagnosis, mechanisms, and risk for recurrence in siblings. Am J Respir Crit Care Med. 2001;164(3):346–357.

28. Patterson K. Crucial Conversations : Tools for Talking When Stakes Are High. New York: McGraw-Hill; 2002.

Chapter 9

Resuscitation, Family Presence, and Last Hours of Living

Eric Bryant, MD, FACEP

Cardiopulmonary Resuscitation and Prognosis in Advanced Illness

Interpreting cardiac arrest survival data can be challenging, but it is clear that cardiopulmonary resuscitation (CPR) is a relatively ineffective intervention, with a 7.6% rate of survival-to-discharge for patients with a prehospital cardiac arrest. Outcomes worsen in the setting of a prolonged downtime and for patients who require prolonged CPR before return of spontaneous circulation.[1]

In the inpatient setting, mortality after cardiac arrest is as high as 83% with a survival rate of less than 7% in patients with sepsis, cancer, uremia, pulmonary embolism (PE), and central nervous system (CNS) disorders. Survival is worse for patients who already require an Intensive Care Unit (ICU) level of care at the time of their arrest.[2] Ewer et al reviewed outcomes of cardiac arrest in 244 patients with cancer for whom resuscitation was attempted. Sixteen patients (6.5%) survived to discharge and all of these had sudden, unanticipated cardiac arrest. Of the patients who had an anticipated cardiac arrest following decline from the progression of their illness, none survived to discharge despite attempts at resuscitation.[3]

In addition, studies reporting survival-to-discharge often do not measure changes in quality of life or functional status, which can be dramatically reduced in survivors of cardiac arrest. Finally, a desire to attempt resuscitation at the time of death also precludes the possibility of a peaceful death at home as emergency medical service (EMS) providers (in the absence of a Do Not Attempt Resuscitation directive) will perform CPR and transport the patient to the emergency department (ED).

Family Presence during Resuscitation

Family presence during resuscitation (FPDR) has been a point of discomfort and debate among medical providers, but studies consistently show that family members often benefit from being present (particularly in the case of parents of pediatric patients). The American Heart Association (AHA) has endorsed family presence in its guidelines.[4] The American College of Emergency

Physicians (ACEP) supports the practice in general, but defers to institutional policies and procedures and emphasizes the need for the care team to be comfortable with family presence. Studies of providers often highlight concerns, including the possibility of interference or misunderstanding, increased litigation due to family distress, and increased stress and anxiety for the ED team. Although these attitudes persist, there is little evidence that FPDR—when handled appropriately—has adverse consequences.[5,6]

Family presence during resuscitation offers a number of potential benefits both for patient and family and for the treatment team. Family presence is likely to be comforting for patients who have some awareness, and it allows family to be with a dying patient while they are still alive. It can help family members understand the gravity of a patient's condition and see that the staff are doing all they can. Seeing the trauma involved in resuscitation can ease their uncertainty about stopping when death is inevitable. This can ease guilt and help provide closure. For the treatment team, family can provide important information about the patient's illness and care preferences, and they can support decision-making. They also serve as a reminder of the patient's individuality and personhood, which can get lost in the mechanics of resuscitation.

If FPDR is to be implemented, a preplanned and structured approach is important to ensure patient safety and family support. The following is a suggested protocol:

Assign a facilitator

Assign an adequately trained staff member to determine whether FDPR is appropriate and coordinate the family presence. First, the medical team must agree to FPDR. Second, the patient, if able, must consent. Third, the facilitator should screen family for appropriateness (to ensure that family members are age-appropriate, calm enough to be present, and not intoxicated or disruptive). Family members should also be supported in their decision not to be present during resuscitation. The number of family members should be limited to one or two, and ideally would include a patient's medical proxy.

Prepare the family

The facilitator should establish ground rules regarding family conduct during attempted resuscitation. In addition, the facilitator should prepare the family for what to expect regarding the patient's appearance, procedures taking place, presence of blood, and the role of various providers in the room.

Attend to the family

The facilitator's role is to attend to the family, and particularly for medically trained personnel, not to be directly involved in patient care. They should answer questions and provide emotional support, but also be prepared to lead family members out of the room if they become overwhelmed or disruptive to the care team.

Stopping

The facilitator can communicate family wishes to the treatment team. If a legal decision-maker is present among the family members, that individual can request that limits be placed on resuscitation efforts. If the family members present are not the legal decision makers, they can still provide guidance to the treating physician, who must judge the medical appropriateness of continuing or ending resuscitation efforts.

Withholding or Withdrawing Nonbeneficial Life-sustaining Interventions

An important skill for the emergency clinician treating dying patients who present to the ED is appropriately withholding or withdrawing interventions such as cardiopulmonary resuscitation, ventilator support, and artificial nutrition and hydration. A key challenge in emergency medicine practice is the information deficit often present when a critically ill patient arrives. Ethics policy statements generally state that absent clear direction to the contrary (from the patient, designated decision-maker, or advance directive), life-prolonging interventions should not be withheld. The consequence of not trying is irreversible, death. Yet when there is a clear directive or request to not have resuscitation, many emergency providers are uncomfortable as most do not have significant experience managing a peaceful death in the ED.[7] But a default setting to perform resuscitation creates the need for clinicians to be able to skillfully and comfortably withdraw unwanted treatments should more information come to light. Such a situation can cause even more discomfort for some providers despite widespread support for the practice in professional organization policy statements and the medical ethics literature.

Cardiopulmonary Resuscitation

Cardiopulmonary Resuscitation (CPR) is a set of interventions intended to reverse the dying process. It includes airway management and ventilation, chest compressions, electrocardioversion, rhythm control, and blood pressure support. It also includes first-responder and bystander interventions taught in a basic life-support class and more advanced interventions included in Advanced Cardiac Life Support. It is often (and inappropriately) presented to patients and families as a menu of choices when in fact, to be effective it needs to be executed as a complete and deliberate package. As discussed above, even when done quickly and correctly average outcomes are not good, but CPR can prove lifesaving and provide an important bridge to definitive therapy for patients with acute isolated conditions such as drowning, electrical injury, or acute myocardial infarction. For patients with multiple medical problems and advanced illness, however, it is rarely beneficial and carries many adverse consequences, such as interfering with a peaceful, natural death; broken ribs and lung injuries; and survival with severe neurologic sequelae.

Many patients do not want "heroic" measures, but they have not communicated this to others or placed these wishes in writing. Others may want an attempt at resuscitation based on a mistaken understanding of outcomes of resuscitation as portrayed in film or television. With a clearer understanding of the reality of resuscitation they may opt to focus on noninvasive interventions and comfort measures at the end of life. There are certainly patients who prefer an attempt at resuscitation, and even a slim chance of prolonging their lives, over any desire to have a peaceful death. In the absence of a signed order or directive to withhold CPR, resuscitation attempts are mandated at the time of death. Each state has a standardized DNR/DNAR directive for out-of-hospital cardiac arrest, and institutions have their own forms for documenting these orders.

Cardiopulmonary resuscitation already under way can be withdrawn when it is clear that the patient will not recover. There are a number of predictors and standards for making the medical determination that continued CPR is not indicated. The other main reason to stop CPR, particularly in patients with advanced illness, is when a decision-maker arrives or an advance directive is located that requests no attempt at resuscitation. As discussed above, family presence during resuscitation can be helpful both to clarify patient wishes and to facilitate a decision to stop CPR.

Intubation and Artificial Ventilation

Although CPR and intubation overlap with artificial ventilation, and preferences exist regarding how one may influence the other, it is worthwhile to maintain a distinction when discussing these interventions. Without airway control and breathing support, cardiopulmonary resuscitation does not work and "partial codes" that exclude them are not medically sound. Aside from cardiopulmonary support, there are numerous reasons to secure an airway and provide ventilator support. These include an acute mental status change from trauma or overdose, a potentially reversible pulmonary process such as pneumonia or edema, or as a part of general anesthesia for major surgery. Intubation and ventilation can be effective therapies to support a patient with a reversible condition to allow time for treatments to take effect.

Although intubation and ventilation almost always occur in the setting of CPR and patients will initially be on a ventilator if they survive a cardiac arrest, intubation and ventilator support are also treatments for impending respiratory failure due to acute illness, such as pneumonia. They also are used to treat an exacerbation of a chronic illness, such as chronic obstructive pulmonary disease (COPD), congestive heart failure (CHF), or cancer. Many patients with these illnesses have experienced being on a ventilator. For some this experience was very uncomfortable and frightening and they do not want to repeat it. Others have seen loved ones on a ventilator and do not want to find themselves in a similar position. The discomfort of an endotracheal tube, the dependence on a "machine," the need for restraints and loss of control all can create significant distress for frail, chronically ill patients. It is quite reasonable that some patients, while wanting a peaceful death and no attempt at resuscitation in their dying moments, would want a time-limited trial of airway and ventilation support in the setting of an acute illness. Others want to be quite clear that they would never want such interventions even if death would result.

Withdrawing ventilator support is a complex subject that raises ethical, emotional, and practical concerns. Patients often present to the ED in extremis and have been intubated by an EMS provider prior to arrival or are intubated during their first moments in the ED. It is not infrequent that new information from family members, a legal decision-maker, or a previously overlooked advance directive reveal that the patient did not want intubation specifically or resuscitation in general. A second common scenario is that the ED workup of an intubated patient reveals a devastating condition such as a large subarachnoid hemorrhage or a ruptured aortic aneurysm. Particularly in chronically ill elderly patients, family or caregivers may want to allow a peaceful death without further invasive care. The usual ED practice would be to admit the patient to the ICU for extubation and terminal care. There are downsides to this approach in that it delays providing a patient with their desired care, thereby prolonging their suffering; it also uses limited resources (ICU bed, nursing, respiratory therapist, and other staff time). There are instances where a brief delay can be beneficial to allow family time to gather. It is critical to provide adequate analgesia and sedation to avoid patient suffering during any delay.

A poorly managed extubation can be cruel for the patient and can lead to prolonged distress and guilt for family members. Providers should follow a standardized protocol to be sure that important steps are not missed, that symptoms are well-palliated, and that family members are supported. Table 9.1 summarizes the key steps to a palliative extubation.

Artificial Nutrition and Hydration

In a normal state of health, hunger and thirst are familiar discomforts and it is reasonable for families to fear that a patient unable to eat or drink is suffering as a result. Many patients with long-term feeding tubes present to the ED with complications such as a blocked displaced tube or an infected tube site. Unlike withholding or withdrawing CPR or ventilator support, a situation where death may follow quickly, a decision to withhold or stop enteral or parenteral nutrition, or even hydration, would not have immediate consequences. It might not seem an important issue in the ED when a patient is going to be admitted to the hospital. However, facilitating decisions about artificial nutrition and hydration (ANH) in the ED can impact a patient's course, particularly when the plan is to discharge to home or a long-term care facility. Although ANH can facilitate recovery and/or prolong life in patients with a reversible process, a mechanical obstruction and in some progressive neurologic disorders such as ALS, in chronically ill, frail elderly patients there is little evidence to support its use.

In approaching a decision about ANH the following questions should be considered:

1. Is the lack of eating and drinking mechanical or functional in origin?
2. If functional, is the disease process reversible?
3. Can the body physiologically tolerate nutrition and hydration, or will it contribute to worsening symptoms such as abdominal discomfort, diarrhea, regurgitation, or third-spacing?
4. Overall, will the patient benefit or be burdened by efforts to provide nutrition or hydration?

Antibiotics

Even treating an "easily reversible" process, such as a pneumonia or urinary tract infection (UTI), may not confer a benefit if a patient does not desire life

Table 9.1 Key Steps to Palliative Extubation	
Before Ventilator Withdrawal	
I. Prepare patient and family	1. Set the stage
	2. Establish preference regarding consciousness
	3. Set expectations
	4. Encourage touch and interactions
	5. Explain uncertainty after withdrawal
	6. Establish DNR status
II. Prepare the ED team	1. Pre-team to discuss plan of care
	2. Review plans for symptom control (dyspnea, anxiety, secretions) with appropriate orders. Have medications at bedside prior to withdrawal
Four Steps to Withdraw	
I. Attend to the setting	1. Physician should turn off alarms
	2. Remove restraints and other unnecessary tubes/ devices
	3. Ensure enough room for family
	4. Allow family to touch, hold patient
	5. Maintain IV access for symptom management
II. Extubation	1. Control symptoms prior to extubation
	2. Set FiO2 to 21 percent
	3. Observe patient, control symptoms
	4. Deflate ETT cuff, turn off ventilator
	5. Remove tube beneath a clean towel and gently clear secretions
III. Support	1. Invite family to touch the patient
	2. Clinician to remain nearby to clear secretions, support family, and continue to manage symptoms/ signs of distress
IV. After-Death Care	1. Encourage family to take the time they need with the patient
	2. Inform of next steps
	3. Offer acute grief support
	4. Offer follow-up bereavement support

prolongation. Infection is a common proximal cause of death in patients with advanced illness and can be a means to die peacefully. While seemingly innocuous (compared to CPR or an endotracheal tube), antibiotics come with some degree of burden, whether that be the need to maintain intravenous access, additional pills that may be difficult to swallow, unpleasant side effects such as nausea or diarrhea, or further complications such as *Clostridium difficile* colitis or fungal infections.

Care of the Actively Dying Patient Recognition

Recognizing that a patient is actively dying may be difficult for the emergency clinician who typically uses a "snapshot approach" to care for patients. Carefully listening for historical clues, most often given by family members or other caregivers, is imperative in order to recognize that a patient may have hours to days. Table 9.2 summarizes key historical and physical findings of patients who are on a terminal illness trajectory at the end of life.[8] This recognition may result in the ability to make a hospice referral or admit to another palliative care setting versus other hospital-based settings that would be less than ideal.

Environment

A key concept in palliative care teaching is to never say "withdraw care." In the last hours of life, many practices can provide comfort to the patient and support to family and friends. Many of the normal features of ED care offer no benefit or can distract from the needs of the dying patient. It is appropriate to discontinue noncomfort measures, such as cardiac and pulse oximetry monitors (or at least turn off alarms), routine vitals, phlebotomy, and diagnostics such as labs and X-rays. Importantly, patients with automatic internal cardiac defibrillators (AICDs) should have the defibrillator function deactivated (with appropriate explanations to family members) so that patients do not experience shocks in their final moments. While not always possible, the patient should be in a quiet

Table 9.2 Signs of Active Dying on a Terminal Illness Trajectory	
Sign	**Examples**
Decreasing level of consciousness	Increasing drowsiness
	Difficulty awakening
	Unresponsive to verbal or tactile stimuli
Decreasing ability to communicate	Difficulty finding words
	Monosyllabic words, short sentences
	Delayed or inappropriate responses
	Verbally unresponsive
Terminal delirium	Early signs of cognitive failure (e.g., day-night reversal)
	Agitation, restlessness
	Purposeless, repetitious movements
	Moaning, groaning
Respiratory dysfunction	Change in ventilatory rate—increasing first, then slowing decreasing tidal volume
	Abnormal breathing patterns—apnea,
	Cheyne-Stokes respirations, agonal breaths
Loss of ability to swallow	Dysphagia, coughing, choking
	Loss of gag reflex
	Buildup of oral and tracheal secretions
	Gurgling
Loss of sphincter control	Incontinence of urine or bowels
	Maceration of skin
	Perineal candidiasis
Pain	Facial grimacing
	Tension in forehead; between eyebrows
Loss of ability to close eyes	Eyelids not closed
	Whites of eyes showing (with or without pupils visible)

room with door, soft lighting (not dark), and chairs for loved ones. A chaplain or other appropriate staff member should be available to provide support and assist with final arrangements after the patient has died.

A useful tool is a preformatted comfort-care order set that reminds the care team about tasks not often performed in the ED, as well as communicates to the patient and family that care and support are being refocused, rather than "stopped" or "withdrawn." A printed information sheet describing the normal and expected signs of dying can be an additional resource. Such information can be helpful both for family and for care-team members who may regard death in the ED as something to be aggressively resisted and a failure when it occurs.

Symptom Control

Symptom management in patients who are actively dying generally follows the same principles as earlier in the course of a patient's illness (see chapters 5–7) with several additional considerations.

Secretions

A patient's inability to manage their secretions is a common finding in the final hours to days of life. (See Table 9.3.) While generally not uncomfortable for the patient, the noisy "death rattle" can be upsetting to family members. Secretions can be managed with anticholinergic agents. Glycopyrrolate given intravenously or subcutaneously is a good first choice for management of secretions because it takes effect quickly, is particularly effective, and does not cross the blood-brain barrier.

Transdermal scopolamine is frequently used for secretions, but is not a good choice when other alternatives are available. It can take 24 hours to reach steady-state and crosses the blood-brain barrier, contributing to delirium and sedation. Among other alternatives, atropine, for instance, also crosses the blood-brain barrier but is more rapid in onset. It can be delivered by placing 1% ophthalmic drops sublingually.[9]

Dry mouth

Conversely patients often have dry mouth and request water. Oral fluids in this setting can lead to choking and aspiration, distressing to the patient and

Table 9.3 Medications for terminal secretions				
Drug	**Trade Name**	**Route**	**Starting Dose**	**Onset**
scopolamine (hyoscine) hydrobromide	Transderm Scop	Patch	One 1.5mg patch	~12 h (24 h to steady state)
hyoscyamine	Levsin	PO,SL	0.125mg	30min
glycopyrrolate	Robinul	PO	0.2mg	30min
glycopyrrolate	Robinul	SubQ, IV	0.1mg	1min
atropine sulfate	Atropine	SubQ, IV	0.1mg	1min
atropine sulfate	multiple	Sublingual	1gtt (1% opth. soln)	30min

the family. There may be a temptation to give IV fluids "for comfort," but this is based on the misunderstanding that IV hydration relieves thirst. Intravenous hydration in this setting generally leads to third-spacing, which can worsen secretions, dyspnea, and abdominal discomfort. The treatment for dry mouth and thirst at the final hours to days of life is mouth care, including moisturizing agents and swabs dipped in cold water.

Agitation
Although haloperidol and chlorpromazine are first-line agents in the management of delirium in the palliative care setting, patients often experience significant agitation at the end of life. This distressing complication can lead to a "bad death" for the patient and prolonged distress for surviving family members. Benzodiazepines such as lorazepam or midazolam are recommended as first-line treatments in the management of hyperactive terminal delirium.

Opioid toxicity
It is very important not to undertreat pain or make significant changes in an otherwise effective analgesic regimen in a patient who is actively dying. That said, as a patient nears the end of life they often will have a decrease in renal function and urine output. In this setting, metabolites of certain opioids, particularly the M3G metabolite of morphine, can accumulate and cause neuroexcitation. This is a form of toxicity that is to be distinguished from more common opioid side effects such as constipation, nausea, sedation, or respiratory depression. Opioid-induced neuroexcitation can manifest as tremors or myoclonic jerks or lead to seizures. If evidence of toxicity exists, patients on an opioid infusion who are actively dying, and who have evidence of decreased urine output, may need to have the basal rate decreased or even held while continuing as-needed bolus doses. The analgesic (and nontoxic) metabolite M6G is also retained in renal failure and its presence can mitigate the decrease in opioid dosing. If a patient cannot tolerate the decrease in opioid in the face of toxicity, and the prognosis is too short to attempt a rotation to an alternative with a lower risk of toxicity such as fentanyl or methadone, then a benzodiazepine can be used to palliate the symptoms of opioid toxicity.

References

1. Sasson C, Rogers MA, Dahl J, Kellermann AL. Predictors of survival from out-of-hospital cardiac arrest: a systematic review and meta-analysis. *Circulation.* 2010;3:63–81.

2. Peberdy MA, Kaye W, Ornato JP, et al. Cardiopulmonary resuscitation of adults in the hospital: a report of 14720 cardiac arrests from the national registry of cardiopulmonary resuscitation. *Resuscitation.* 2003;58:297–308.

3. Ewer MS, Kish SK, Martin CG, Price KJ, Feeley TW. Characteristics of cardiac arrest in cancer patients as a predictor of survival after cardiopulmonary resuscitation. *Cancer.* 2001;92:1905–1912.

4. Morrison LJ, Kierzek G, Diekema DS, et al. Part 3: Ethics: 2010 American Heart Association guidelines for cardiopulmonary resuscitation and emergency cardiovascular care. *Circulation.* 2010;122:S665–S675.

5. Duran CR, Oman K, Abel JJ, Koziel VM, Szymanski D. Attitudes toward and beliefs about family presence: a survey of healthcare providers, patients' families, and patients. *Am J Crit Care.* 2007;16(3):270–279.

6. Dudley NC, Hansen KW, Furnival RA, Donaldson AE, Van Wagenen KL, Scaife ER. The effect of family presence on the efficiency of pediatric trauma resuscitations. *Ann Emerg Med.* 2009;53:777–784.

7. Smith AK, Fisher J, Schonberg MA, et al. Am I doing the right thing? Provider perspectives on improving palliative care in the emergency department. *Ann Emerg Med.* 2009;54:86–93, 93.E1.

8. Ferris D. Last hours of living. Clin Geriatr Med. 2004;20(4):641–67, vi.

9. Brickel K, Arnold R. #109 Death Rattle and Oral Secretions. 2nd ed. http://www.eperc.mcw.edu/EPERC/FastFactsIndex/ff_109.htm. Accessed October 3, 2012.

Chapter 10

Hospice Care

Sangeeta Lamba, MD

Introduction

Emergency clinicians often care for patients with a terminal life-limiting illness who are receiving hospice care, and many more patients who may be in need of and eligible for such care.[1-5] In many countries, the terms palliative care and hospice care may often be used synonymously, but it is important to note that in the United States there is a distinction between these terms based on prognosis.[6] Palliative care eligibility is based on the needs of the patient (ideal onset at the time of diagnosis of a severe life-limiting disease such as cancer). On the other hand, hospice care eligibility is primarily based on a prognosis of living 6 months or less.[1,2,6] Emergency clinicians familiar with the hospice model may be better able to guide patients and caregivers at end-of-life.[1-5] This chapter first reviews the hospice care service model and then discusses who may qualify for hospice; common emergency presentations in patients under hospice care; and finally outlines a stepwise approach to initiating a new referral to hospice care from the emergency department (ED).

Understanding Hospice Care

The word hospice originates from the Latin word "*hospitium*," a rest-house for weary and tired travelers. Dr. Cicely Saunders began the modern hospice movement during the 1960s, when she established St. Christopher's Hospice near London, which provided comprehensive palliative care for dying patients.[7] Her visit to Yale added impetus to the idea of specialized care for the dying and led to the establishment of the first hospice in the United States in New Haven, Connecticut in 1974.[8] Currently, the hospice care model is based on provision of quality, compassionate care for those facing a severe life-limiting illness and it uses a team-oriented, multidisciplinary approach to medical care, pain management, and emotional/spiritual support that is tailored to fit the patient's and family's needs.[1,7,8] Hospice is therefore not a place, but a care system where emphasis is on quality of life and "living until you die."[8-10]

Eligibility

In the United States, hospice services are delivered in a model that was established by a statute in Medicare (1982) and is now followed by most insurers.[11] Under the Medicare Hospice Benefit, patients are eligible for hospice services if they have a prognosis of 6 months or less if their disease runs its usual course (because some patients may outlive this prognosis).[11-15] In general, for a patient to receive hospice care, two physicians (an attending physician and the hospice medical director) certify that to the best of their judgment, the patient is terminally ill and more likely than not, to die within 6 months if the disease runs its normal course; *and* the patient/family consents to the hospice philosophy of a comfort care approach with respect to their terminal illness, forgoing most therapies that have a curative intent.[11–16] There is no penalty if a patient survives longer. Patients may become ineligible for hospice services with improvement in their health status (so-called hospice graduate), but may re-enroll if their clinical condition declines. Patients may have any diagnosis to qualify for hospice care, and noncancer primary diagnoses now comprise greater than 58% of all admissions to hospice.[10] To assist physicians in prognostication and assessment of eligibility for hospice, broad guidelines for many cancer and noncancer-related conditions exist (Table 10.1).[12,13] It is important to note however, that these are

Table 10.1 General Hospice Eligibility Guidelines	
General Guidelines	Progression of life-limiting disease as documented by: • Decline in clinical status—recurrent infections, intractable pain or vomiting/diarrhea, dysphagia • Multiple hospital admissions or emergency department (ED) visits • Decline in functional status—dependence on assistance with activities of daily living • Impaired nutritional status—weight loss 10% over past 6 months, serum albumin < 2.5 g/L • Disease specific markers—physical examination, labs, prior imaging
Disease Specific General Guidelines	
Oncologic	• Disease with distant metastases at presentation *or* • Progression from an earlier stage of disease to metastatic disease with either: (1) a continued decline in spite of therapy; and/or (2) patient declines further disease directed therapy
Cardiac	• Congestive heart failure (CHF) symptoms at rest (New York Hospital Association [NYHA] Classification IV) • Must be optimally treated with diuretics and after-load reduction • The following help predict increased mortality: symptomatic supraventricular or ventricular arrhythmias, prior cardiac arrest, unexplained syncope, cardiogenic shock • An ejection fraction of 20% or less is helpful, but not required
Pulmonary	• Disabling dyspnea at rest; unresponsive to treatment • Progressive disease —declining FEV1 (> 40 mL/year) or increased ED visits/hospitalizations • Cor pulmonale or right-heart failure (not due to valve disease or left-heart failure) • Hypoxemia at rest (PaO2 < 55 mm Hg or sat < 88% on supplemental O2) • Hypercapnea (PaCO2 > 50 mm Hg) (records within last 3 months) • Resting tachycardia

(continued)

Table 10.1	Continued
Dementia	1. Patients with all the following characteristics:
	• Stage seven or beyond according to the Functional Assessment Staging Scale
	• Unable to ambulate, dress, or bathe without assistance
	• Urinary and fecal incontinence, intermittent or constant
	• No consistently meaningful verbal communication: limited to six or fewer intelligible words.
	2. Presence of co-morbid conditions associated with decreased survival, such as: aspiration, pyelonephritis, septicemia, pressure ulcers (stage 3–4), fever despite antibiotics.
	3. Nutritional impairment
	• If patient has G-tube, nutritional impairment with weight loss > 10% over 6 months, serum albumin < 2.5 g/L
	• In the absence of G-tube, decreased oral intake
Liver	• Not a transplant candidate
	• Impaired synthetic function: Albumin < 2.5 g/L and international normalized ratio (INR) > 1.5
	• Ascites despite maximum diuretics
	• Spontaneous bacterial peritonitis
	• Hepatorenal syndrome
	• Hepatic encephalopathy despite management
	• Recurrent variceal bleeding
Renal	• Creatinine clearance < 10cc/min (< 15 if diabetic) and serum creatinine > 8 (> 6 if diabetic)
	• Signs or symptoms associated with uremia—hyperkalemia, pericarditis
	• Oliguria
	• Intractable fluid overload
	• Not on, or refusing, dialysis
HIV	CD4 of < 25 despite anti-retroviral therapy, decreased functional status plus one of the following;
	• Central nervous system (CNS) lymphoma
	• Persistent wasting
	• Mycobacterium avium complex bacteremia
	• Progressive multifocal leukoencephalopathy
	• Visceral Kaposi's or systemic lymphoma resistant to chemotherapy
	• Cryptosporidium or Toxoplasmosis resistant to therapy

Adapted from the Centers for Medicare and Medicaid Services—Medicare coverage database. LCD (Local Coverage Determination) for Hospice-Determining Terminal Status (L25678).[12] Available at: http://www. cms.gov/mcd/viewlcd.asp?lcd_id=25678&lcd_version=27&show=all#top

not hard-and-fast rules, and coexisting conditions or a rapid functional decline can outweigh strict adherence to these guidelines.[1,12,13,16]

Underutilization

Studies reveal that patients with a terminal illness often receive poor-quality end-of-life care that is burdened with untreated symptoms, unmet psychosocial needs, and overall low patient and family satisfaction.[6,9,17,18] Studies also demonstrate that hospice programs may improve care provision of physical and psychosocial symptoms, support family/caregiver well-being, assist bereavement outcomes, and increase patient, family, and physician satisfaction.[6,14,20–22] Hospice care has also been associated with reductions in total healthcare expenditure.[14,23–25] A recent analysis found that the costs of care for patients with cancer who dis-enrolled from hospice were nearly five times higher than those for patients who remained with hospice, perhaps due to increased emergency department care and hospitalizations.[26]

Despite demonstrable improvement in the quality of end-of-life care and widespread availability, hospice care remains globally underutilized.[10,16] In 2007, of the total 2.4 million deaths in the United States, 38% of patients received hospice care.[10] When patients receive hospice care, the median length of service is about 20 days, with approximately one-third of patients served receiving hospice care for only 7 days or less, often too late for meaningful payment to end-of-life care.[10] Reasons for late hospice referrals are multifactorial and include both patient- and physician-related barriers. Some of these barriers include reluctance of physicians to prognosticate and communicate the resultant prognosis to their patients; unwillingness of patients or families to accept the terminality of their illness, considering hospice only for those who are imminently dying; and racial as well as ethnic factors.[16,27–30] Patients and families may perceive that choosing hospice care "hastens" death and is equal to "giving up hope." Contrary to this widely held assumption, some evidence now suggests that patients do not have shorter lives as a result of hospice enrollment alone.[31–33] The improvement in psychosocial support, caregiver support, and perhaps the reduction in higher risk medical interventions in those under hospice care may even prolong mean survival in certain patient populations, though more studies still have to establish generalizability of these findings.[31–33]

Scope of Services and Reimbursement

The selected hospice agency becomes the patient's care manager and is paid a per diem rate for all care that is provided to the patient and is related to the primary hospice-certifying diagnosis.[12–14] Hospice care is provided by a multidisciplinary team that includes a physician, nurses, social workers, chaplaincy support, home health aides, volunteers, and therapists. Patients may also keep seeing their own primary care providers for continuity of care. Members of the hospice team meet regularly to set patient care plans, discuss ongoing issues, and make regular visits to assess the patient for needed care and support services. They are on call 24 hours a day, 7 days a week.[10–16] Hospice care plans include the management of pain and other distressing symptoms; provision of symptom- and comfort-related medications, medical supplies, and durable medical equipment; assistance with emotional, psychosocial, and spiritual aspects of dying; caregiver support and guidance on how to care for the patient; speech and physical therapy; short-term inpatient care when symptoms become difficult to manage at home, for those actively dying or when the caregiver needs respite time; and bereavement care to the surviving family and caregivers for 1 year after patient death.[10–16]

Hospice services are fully covered under Medicare, Medicaid, and private insurers. Hospice is responsible for *all* care costs related to the hospice-qualifying diagnosis for which the patient is certified. Because hospice is the care manager, the agency will ask patients/surrogates to call them first before seeking emergency care in order to determine whether the condition is related to the patient's hospice-qualifying diagnosis and whether hospice can manage the crisis without an ED visit. Patients under hospice care may present to the ED for conditions related to or not related to their hospice-qualifying diagnosis, and reimbursement responsibility may therefore vary.[1] For example, when a patient with a hospice-qualifying diagnosis of metastatic breast cancer presents to the ED with a cut to her knee from a minor fall (unrelated to the cancer), the regular insurer is billed and pays for related charges. In contrast, if the same patient presents to the ED for a minor fall and has a pathologic femur fracture, the condition *is* related to the cancer (primary certifying diagnosis), and hospice is held fiscally responsible for ED service charges. The patient also may sometimes be held fiscally responsible for ED charges if they fail to notify hospice of their intent to seek emergency care and the issue could have been resolved easily by the hospice provider.

Discontinuing hospice care

Along with the hospice graduate who leaves hospice care due to an improvement in the underlying condition, patients may decide to opt out of hospice care for a number of other reasons. These may include: (1) patient or surrogates may have difficulty accepting the terminal nature of their illness; (2) they may disagree with the comfort care philosophy and decide to seek care directed at prolonging life that cannot be provided by hospice; (3) they may desire a second opinion of therapeutic, curative options; and (4) they may be dissatisfied with the hospice care model or service.[1] From the hospice agency perspective, a patient may sometimes be discharged from hospice if patient behavior is disruptive, abusive, and uncooperative to the extent that provision of appropriate hospice care is compromised or cannot be provided in a safe environment by the healthcare provider.

Emergency department care does not automatically equate to hospice termination.[1,35] Sometimes hospice providers may themselves initiate the call to emergency services for a patient transfer to the ED if hospitalization is indicated and hospice is unable to manage that particular aspect of care.[1] The call to emergency services may also be initiated by hospice providers for a patient with imminent deterioration who has not elected the do-not-resuscitate (DNR) status. Though many hospice patients opt for a DNR status, this is not universally true.[1,17,35,36] End-of-life-preference discussions, including DNR status, are part of ongoing hospice and patient communications, but early in the enrollment phase the patient may not be ready to face such decisions. Other patients may object to DNR due to religious or philosophical reasons. It is therefore important for the ED clinician to recognize that designation of DNR is *not* a prerequisite for hospice enrollment and also not a reason to terminate hospice care.[1,35]

Emergency Department Management of Patients Under Hospice Care

Recent studies highlight the ambivalence and discomfort that emergency physicians and residents face when treating patients with hospice and palliative needs.[37] These findings are not surprising in a field dedicated to acute management of illness with a focus on resuscitation, stabilization, and life-prolonging measures. The many barriers to optimal ED care at end-of-life may include a cha-otic environment, competing demands, and long wait times, as well as numerous communication-related challenges.[1–5,37] Emergency department providers may face distress and conflict when patients' wishes or written advance directives conflict with the wishes of family.[37] Resident trainees in one study expressed concern about inadequacy in pain management training and also expressed re-gret that dying patients they had cared for had received suboptimal pain manage-ment.[37] Emergency Medicine literature is now addressing this gap and attempting to define the best ways to educate and enhance the generalist-level palliative skills of trainees so that they can rapidly adapt to and switch from an aggressive-to a comfort-care approach at end-of-life, when needed.[1,2,38,39]

Emergency department providers should not assume that arrival in the ED by a hospice patient equates to a desire for aggressive and life-prolonging treatment.[1,35] Some patients will activate a call to emergency services as an ingrained "learned behavior" that is an automatic response to any perceived acute distress.[1] Therefore, at the time of ED arrival, an assessment is needed to understand the concerns that prompted a shift in care goals or to identify the underlying reason that triggered the ED visit. Frequently such requests arise from fear about the dying process, guilt about prior medical decisions to limit life-prolonging treatments, or a conflict in end-of-life decision-making with a family member.[1,35,40] Some common triggers for an ED visit are listed in Table 10.2.[1,35,40] A multidisciplinary approach with involvement of hospice, so-cial services, and palliative team members (if available) may assist in providing optimal care for ED patients under hospice care.

A general approach to ED care of the hospice patient is outlined in Table 10.3. It is important to note that early involvement of hospice and pri-mary care providers, as well as effective communication regarding plans of care

---

Table 10.2 Triggers for a Hospice Patient to Seek an Emergency Department Visit

Common Triggers for an ED Visit:

Patient and caregiver factors

1. Poor symptom control (especially pain and dyspnea)
2. Malfunction or loss of support devices (tracheostomy or gastrostomy tube)
3. Stress, fear, and inability to cope with impending loss of life
4. Conflict regarding life-prolonging treatments (either begun in past and discontinued, e.g., chemotherapy; or never started, e.g., renal dialysis)
5. Competing philosophies of approach to care between caregiver and patient
6. Caregiver fatigue
7. Automatic ingrained response to perceived distress

Hospice factors

8. Failure or inability to communicate with or address patient needs in a timely manner
9. Equipment failure unable to be repaired in a timely manner (e.g., home oxygen or nebulizer machine)
10. Call initiated by hospice (unable to provide that aspect of care or patient is a "full code")

Adapted from *Fast Fact # 246* with permission[35]

Table 10.3 General Management Guidelines When Providing Emergency Department Care for a Patient

Notify hospice staff as soon as possible	Not only is hospice legally/financially responsible for the patient's plan of care/medical costs related to the terminal illness, they have an ongoing understanding of patient related issues.
Determine the trigger	Pay attention to not only the distressing signs and symptoms but also the emotional and psycho-social issues. Involve social service/chaplaincy and palliative care team early, if needs are identified.
Treat distressing symptoms	*See specific symptom treatment guidelines*
If deterioration is imminent	If rapid decisions are needed regarding the use of life-sustaining treatments (e.g., intubation for respiratory failure), a focused discussion around goals of care must occur in the emergency department.
	– Identify the legal decision-maker and review any completed advance directives.
	– Complete rapid goals of care discussion (see chapter....).
	– *Make recommendations* For example, "According to what you want for [the patient], I would/would not recommend..."
If the patient is actively dying	Assess for cultural/spiritual needs; ensure privacy and seek to identify whether there are any preferred locations to which a patient can be safely transferred for the dying process (e.g., back home; to a private hospital room).
Laboratory tests/ diagnostics	These should be limited or withheld until discussion with the patient's hospice care team. Testing should be based on patient-defined goals of care.
	Generally, low-burden, noninvasive methods, which may reveal reversible pathology or clarify prognosis should be used first.
Therapeutic modalities	Therapy should be based on patient-defined goals of care. Automatic "ED algorithms" (e.g., antibiotics for pneumonia) should only be used if they meet patient goals of care.
Disposition	Should be planned *after* discussion with hospice staff and be based on the patient's goals. Returning home or a direct admission to an inpatient hospice facility may be the best disposition rather than hospital admission. If patient wishes for a home setting, hospices may be able to arrange 24h support for those with difficult to manage symptoms.
Notify the patient or surrogate and hospice	The inpatient palliative care service (if available) and hospice should be notified if the patient is to be admitted to the hospital. Patient and caregiver should be aware of next steps of plan (discharge home on adjusted pain medication, inpatient hospice care etc.)

Adapted from *Fast Fact # 246* with permission[35]

and disposition is essential.[1,35,41–43] Often, patients under hospice present to the ED with life-threatening crisis events and questions about resuscitation and the use of life-sustaining interventions frequently arise.[1,35,37,43,44] The process of delineating patient wishes in this setting is difficult because in a crisis situation the patient is often unable to verbalize and surrogates may not be easily accessible. In addition, there are other challenges to implementation of pre-existing advance planning documents. These may include an unanticipated change in health status, interfamily conflicts, and issues with institutional protocols.[1,37] Therefore, discussion of relevant decisions needs to occur real-time in the ED and rapid advance-care planning and delineation of goals of care is usually necessary.[1,35,45,46] It is best not to isolate discussions about cardiopulmonary resuscitation and DNR but rather make recommendations in a general context based on overall patient wishes and goals.[46] It is also important to highlight ongoing clinician availability and emphasize nonabandonment.[43,47]

Common Presentations

Patients under hospice care may present to the ED for terminal illness-related or unrelated reasons. Some of the common ED presentations of patients under hospice care include control of severe pain, dyspnea, acute management of fever/infections, and provision of care for the imminently dying patient.[1,2,4,9,40]

Uncontrolled pain at the end of life is particularly important to address in those with advanced malignancy because these patients may have a high burden of pain, are often opiate tolerant, and may be receiving high doses of opioids.[48] Many resources, especially on the Web are easily available to aid the ED clinician in managing severe pain in such opioid-tolerant patients.[49–53] It is important to remember that there is no ceiling or maximal recommended dose and during the hospital and ED stay the patient will likely need a "fixed dose schedule" in addition to the more familiar "as needed" or PRN opioid orders for acute pain.[48–51]

Because it provokes anxiety in patients and caregivers, *respiratory distress* is another common end-of-life presentation in hospice patients.[1,40,44,54] Evaluation and management of dyspnea is, again, dependent on understanding where the patient is in the dying trajectory and is based on patient-identified goals of care.[1,54] If goals of care are yet to be determined, or the patient is not in the terminal stages of his/her illness trajectory, a rapid evaluation to determine easily reversible causes, such as anemia and pleural effusion, may be warranted using the least invasive diagnostic tests first (e.g., chest radiograph and pulse oximeter). Terminal dyspnea in an actively dying patient, however, may be best addressed with a comfort-care approach.[55] Family reassurance, in addition to noninvasive measures such as oxygen, upright positioning, and a fan to blow cool air on the face, may help.[1,55] Opioids remain the first-line agents to break the vicious cycle of anxiety-dyspnea, and if needed, benzodiazepines may be added for patient comfort.[56] Noninvasive ventilation may provide a bridge that allows time to clarify life-extending therapies.[1,54]

Fever and infections in hospice patients are often reasons for presenting to the ED.[1,40] Again, management and assessment is based on understanding where the patient is in the dying trajectory and should also be based on patient-identified goals of care. Antibiotics, especially oral, are often used to address symptoms and improve quality of life for hospice patients (as in urinary tract infection or pneumonia). Often, patients also are able to go home with hospice providing intravenous antibiotics, if needed. Real-time discussions about early goal-directed therapy, and invasive or intensive care management, are based on overall patient goals of care and may need to be arbitrated on a case-by-case basis.

Imminently dying hospice patients often present to the ED due to caregiver distress and lack of coping with impending loss of life.[1,35,44,47] It is important to note that decreased oral intake and worsening mentation are to be expected in a natural death. Therefore, the automatic response to start intravenous hydration may not always be suitable or desired in the setting of this final dying process. Prehospital emergency providers called in this setting should always ask for any advance care plan, and honor any written directives that can be identified on scene and are recognized in provider protocols. In many situations where directives are not available, a titrated therapeutic approach may include use of noninvasive supportive care first (e.g., oxygen, noninvasive ventilation) to bridge arrival to ED or until goals are clarified. However, full prehospital resuscitation is often instituted as a 'default' response when emergency providers are faced with a life-threatening crisis in the setting of unclear and unavailable directives. If such a patient presents to the ED, and further discussions reveal that life-support interventions were "unwanted" or are no longer desired, the ED clinician should be prepared to offer withdrawal of life-prolonging measures.[1] The most commonly withdrawn therapy in dying patients is mechanical ventilation, followed by vasoactive drugs.[57] Several commonly used algorithms for the medical management of withdrawal of ventilator support exist and most institutions have written protocols for clinician guidance.[58,59] Family or surrogates should be prepared for withdrawal of the ventilator, and care must be taken to inform them that the patient may not die immediately and may in fact survive for hours to days after removal.[60,61] A quiet, private setting, chaplaincy (if desired), and palliative team support for family (if available) is optimal. Care must be taken to provide adequate patient sedation for comfort during the withdrawal process and the clinician should be readily available to address family concerns and questions.[61,62]

Initiating New Hospice Referrals from the Emergency Department

Patients with an end-stage terminal illness often present to the ED with a crisis event.[1,2,4,9,40,43,44] In eligible patients (refer to Table 10.1), this crisis visit may present a unique opportunity to establish patient goals of care. In those who seek a comfort-care-based approach, the ED visit may therefore often present the opportunity to initiate hospice care discussions.[63–64] Generally this means a patient wants medical treatments and other support aimed at alleviating symptoms and maintaining quality of life, without life-prolongation. Patients may enroll in hospice care if their *preeminent* care goal is the relief of symptoms, even if they are not entirely certain they want to completely discontinue life-prolonging therapies, as long as the hospice agency is able to accommodate those wishes.[64] Disposition to hospice care in eligible patients may also reduce length of hospital stay, reduce ED visits at the end of life, and enhance bereavement care in survivors with improved patient and caregiver satisfaction.[6,40] An up-to-date listing of available community resources and a stepwise approach may assist the new hospice referral process from the ED, as outlined in Table 10.4.[64,65]

Table 10.4 Initiating a Referral to Hospice Care from the Emergency Department

1. Assess eligibility for Medicare Hospice Benefit	– This essentially means that the patient has a prognosis that is 6 months or less if his/her disease runs its expected course. – Broad guidelines for hospice eligibility exist (see table 10.1). – A useful starting point is to ask yourself, *"Would I be surprised if this patient died within the next 6 months?"*
2. Discuss hospice as a disposition plan with the patient's physician	– Contact the patient's personal physician; discuss the current condition, prognosis, and prior goals of care conversations. – Ask if the physician is willing to be the following physician of record for hospice.
3. Assess whether the patient's goals are consistent with hospice care	These four questions may help start the discussion to elicit whether the patient/family is/are psychologically ready to accept hospice. • *"What have you been told about the status of your illness and what the future holds?"* • *"Has anyone talked to you about your prognosis; how much time you likely have?"* • *"Are there plans for new treatments designed to help you extend your life?"* • *"Has anyone discussed hospice services with you? What do you know about hospice?"*
4. Introduce hospice to the patient and family or surrogates	– Discuss the core aspects of hospice and how features can help the patient (e.g., 24/7 on-call assistance, home visits for symptom management, and emotional and chaplaincy support). – Address concerns and clarify misconceptions. – Phrase your recommendation for hospice care in positive language, grounded in the patient's own care goals. *"I think the best way to help you stay at home, avoid the hospital, and stay as fit as possible for whatever time you have left is to receive hospice care at your home...."*

5. Make a referral

– Call a hospice agency and anticipate following questions:
- What is the terminal illness? Who will be the following physician? (Step 2)
- What equipment will be needed immediately (e.g., home oxygen)? Is there a caregiver at home?
- Code status. Patients cannot be denied hospice enrollment if "full code," however the hospice team should be aware that code status needs to be addressed.

6. Write orders

Sample ED Initiated Hospice Referral Orders:
- Evaluate and Admit/Enroll _____ in hospice care.
- Terminal Diagnosis: _____.
- Expected Prognosis: Terminal illness with less than 6-month survival likely if disease runs its normal expected course [or more specific if indicated].
- Physician who will follow patient: _____

7. Ensure patient/surrogate understanding and secure the plan.

– Communicate the plan following ED discharge (next steps).
– Provide the name and contact number for the hospice agency.

Adapted from *Fast Fact # 247* with permission[64]

Hospice care usually is provided and set up at the location the patient prefers to call home, either a private residence or long-term care facility. Direct admissions to hospice facilities can occur depending on bed availability and ability of local hospice agencies to arrange an immediate direct facility admission. This is not available in all communities and requires a discussion with the hospice agency. Sometimes a hospice referral may be appropriate, but cannot be arranged in a timely manner from the ED.[64] In this case, if the patient can be cared for at home safely for 1–2 days without extra services, he/she may be discharged home with appropriate prescriptions and care instructions.[64] In most communities, patients can be enrolled in hospice care within 24–48 hours, even on weekends. If a patient cannot be cared for safely at home, observation versus inpatient admission is likely necessary until a safe discharge plan can be social services and palliative care team.[64]

References

1. Lamba S, Quest TE. Hospice care and the Emergency Department: rules, regulations and referrals. *Ann Emerg Med*. 2011;57:282–290.

2. Quest TE http://www.sciencedirect.com/science/article/pii/S019606440 8020581 - cor1, Marco CA, Derse AR. Hospice and palliative medicine: new subspecialty, new opportunities. *Ann Emerg Med*. 2009;54(1):94–102.

3. Chan GK. End-of-life and palliative care in the emergency department: a call for research, education, policy and improved practice in this frontier area. *J Emerg Nurs*. 2006;32(1):101–103.

4. Lamba S, Mosenthal AC. Hospice and palliative medicine; a new subspecialty of emergency medicine. *J Emerg Med*. 2012;43(5):849–853.

5. Chan GK. End-of-life models and emergency department care. *Acad Emerg Med*. 2004;11(1):79–86.

6. Meier DE. Increased access to palliative care and hospice services: opportunities to improve value in health care. *Milbank Q*. 2011;89(3):343–380.

7. Bennahum DA. Hospice and palliative care: concepts and practice. In: Forman W, Kitzes J, Anderson RP, et al, eds. *The Historical Development of Hospice and Palliative Care*. 2nd ed. Sudbury, MA: Jones and Bartlett;2003.

8. Krisman-Scott MA. Origins of hospice in the United States: the care of the dying, 1945–1975. *J Hosp Palliat Nurs*. 2003;5(4):205–210.

9. SUPPORT Principal Investigators. A controlled trial to improve care for seriously ill hospitalized patients. The Study to Understand Prognoses and Preferences for Outcomes and Risks of Treatments (SUPPORT). *JAMA*. 1995;274:1591–1598.

10. National Hospice and Palliative Care Organization. NHPCO facts and figures: hospice care in America. Alexandria, VA: NHPCO; 2008. Available at: http://www.nhpco.org/files/public/Statistics_Research/NHPCO_facts-and-figures_Nov2007.pdf. Accessed January 14, 2012.

11. Hoyer T. A history of the Medicare hospice benefit. *Hospice J*.1998;13:61–69.

12. Centers for Medicare & Medicaid Services, Medicare Coverage Database. LCD (local coverage determination) for hospice: determining terminal status (L25678). Available at: http:// www.cms.gov/mcd/viewlcd.asp?lcd_id_25678&lcd_version_27&show_all#top. Accessed January 13, 2012.

13. Center for Medicare Education. The Medicare hospice benefit. Issue brief. 2001;2:1–6. Available at: http://www.MedicareEd.org. Accessed January 10, 2012.

14. Emanuel EJ, Ash A, Yu W, et al. Managed care, hospice use, site of death, and medical expenditures in the last year of life. *Arch Intern Med.* 2002;162:1722–1728.

15. Harmon D. No time limit on Medicare hospice benefit. *Am J Hospice Palliat Med.* 2005;22:93.

16. Gazelle G. Understanding hospice—an underutilized option for life's final chapter. *N Engl J Med.* 2007;357:321–324.

17. Teno, JM, Clarridge BR, Casey V, et al. Family perspectives on end-of-life care at the last place of care. *JAMA* 2004;291:88–93.

18. Thorpe KE, Howard DH. The rise in spending among Medicare beneficiaries: The role of chronic disease prevalence and changes in treatment intensity. *Health Aff (Millwood).* 2006;25:w378–388.

19. Wright AA, Zhang B, Ray A, et al. Associations between end-of-life discussions, patient mental health, medical care near death, and caregiver bereavement adjustment. *JAMA.* 2008;300:1665–1673.

20. Zhang B, Wright AA, Huskamp HA, et al. Health care costs in the last week of life: Associations with end-of-life conversations. *Arch Intern Med.* 2009;169:480–488.

21. Wright AA, Keating N, Balboni T, Matulonis U, Block S, Prigerson H. Place of death: Correlations with quality of life of patients with cancer and predictors of bereaved caregivers' mental health. *J Clin Oncol.* 2010;28:4457–4464.

22. Ringdal GI, Jordhoy MS, and Kaasa S. Family satisfaction with end-of-life care for cancer patients in a cluster randomized trial. *J Pain Symptom Manage.* 2002:24:53–63.

23. Christakis NA, Iwashyna TJ. The health impact of health care on families: A matched cohort study of hospice use by decedents and mortality outcomes in surviving widowed spouses. *Soc Sci Med.* 2003;57:465–475.

24. Morrison RS, Meier DE. Clinical practice. Palliative care. *N Engl J Med.* 2004;350:2582–2590.

25. Taylor D. Effect of hospice on Medicare and informal care costs: the United States experience. *J Pain Symptom Manage.* 2009;38:110–114.

26. Carlson M, Herrin J, Du Q, et al. Impact of hospice disenrollment on health care use and Medicare expenditures for patients with cancer. *J Clin Oncol.* 2010;28:4371–4375.

27. Teno JM, Shu JE, Casarett D, et al. Timing of referral to hospice and quality of care: length of stay and bereaved family members' perceptions of the timing of hospice referral. *J Pain Symptom Manage.* 2007;34:120–125.

28. Labyak M. Ten myths and facts about hospice care. *Home Healthc Nurse.* 2002;20:148.

29. Quill TE. Is length of stay on hospice a critical quality of care indicator? *J Palliat Med.* 2007;10:290–292.

30. Han B, Remsburg RE, Iwashyna TJ. Differences in hospice use between black and white patients during the period 1992 through 2000. *Med Care.* 2006;44:731–737.

31. Connor SR, Pyenson B, Fitch K, Spence C, Iwasaki K. Comparing hospice and nonhospice patient survival among patients who die within a three-year window. *J Pain Symptom Manage.* 2007;33:238–246.

32. Bakitas M, Lyons K, Hegel M, Balan S, Brokaw F, et al. Effects of a palliative care intervention on clinical outcomes in patients with advanced cancer: The Project ENABLE II randomized controlled trial. *JAMA.* 2009;302:741–749.

33. Temel J, Greer J, Muzikansky A, Gallagher E, Admane S, et al. Early palliative care for patients with metastatic non-small-cell lung cancer. *N Engl J Med.* 2010;363:733–742.

34. Department of Health and Human Services. *Correction to Annual Change in Hospice Payment Rates.* Washington, DC: Department of Health and Human Services; 2009.

35. Lamba S, Quest TE, Weissman DE. Emergency Department management of hospice patients. *Fast Facts and Concepts.* 2011; 246. Available at: http://www.eperc.mcw.edu/EPERC/FastFactsIndex/Documents/ff_246.htm. Last accessed January 16, 2012.

36. Miller SC, Mor V, Wu N, et al. Does receipt of hospice care in nursing homes improve the management of pain at the end of life? *J Am Geriatr Soc.* 2002;50:507–515.

37. Smith AK, Fisher J, Schonberg MA, et al. Am I doing the right thing? Provider perspectives on improving palliative care in the emergency department. *Ann Emerg Med.* 2009.54(1):86–93.

38. Lamba S, Pound A, Rella JR, Compton S. Emergency Medicine resident education in palliative care: a needs assessment. *J Palliat Med.* 2012; 15(5)516–520.

39. Gisondi MA. A case for education in palliative and end-of-life care in emergency medicine. *Acad Emerg Med.* 2009;16:181–183.

40. Barbera L, Taylor C, Dudgeon D. Why do patients with cancer visit the emergency department near the end of life? *CMAJ.* 2010;182(6):563–568.

41. Reeves K. Hospice care in the emergency department. *J Emerg Nurs.* 2008;34:350–351.

42. Reeves K. Hospice care in the emergency department: important things to remember. *J Emerg Nurs.* 2000;26:477–478; quiz 528.

43. Smith AK, Schonberg MA, Fisher J, et al. Emergency Department experiences of acutely symptomatic patients with terminal illness and their family caregivers. *J Pain Symptom Manage..* 2010;39(6):972–981.

44. Grudzen CR, Richardson LD, Morrison M, Cho E, Morrison RS. Palliative care needs of seriously ill, older patients presenting to the emergency department. *Acad Emerg Med.* 2010; 17(11):1253–1257.

45. Stump BF, Klugman CM, Thornton B. Last hours of life: encouraging end-of-life conversations. *J Clin Ethics.* 2008;19:150–159.

46. Von Gunten CF, Weissman DE. Discussing DNR orders—part 1, 2nd ed. *Fast Facts and Concepts.* 2005; fast fact 23. Available at: http://www.eperc.mcw.edu/fastfact/ff_023.htm. Accessed January 4, 2012.

47. Bailey CJ, Murphy R, Porock D. Trajectories of end-of-life care in the Emergency Department. *Ann Emerg Med.* 2011;57:362–369.

48. Desandre PL, Quest TE. Management of cancer-related pain. *Emerg Med Clin North Am.* 2009;27:179–194.

49. Davis MP, Weissman DE, Arnold RM. Opioid dose titration for severe cancer pain: a systematic evidence-based review. *J Palliat Med.* 2004;7:462–468.

50. Arnold R, Weissman DE. Calculating opioid dose conversions #36. *J Palliat Med.* 2003;6:619–620.

51. Weissman DE. Opioid dose escalation. 2nd ed. *Fast Facts and Concepts.* 2005: fast fact 20. Available at: http://www.eperc.mcw.edu/fastfact/ff_020.htm. Accessed January 13, 2012.

52. Pain Task Force, Massachusetts General Hospital. Opioid potency and equianalgesia: critical facts, 2005. Available at: http://www2.massgeneral.org/painrelief/equianalgesia.pdf. Accessed January 16, 2012.

53. End-of-life Palliative Education Research Center. Educational materials and fast facts sections. Available at: http://www.eperc.mcw.edu. Accessed January 11, 2012.

54. LaDuke S. Terminal dyspnea and palliative care. *Am J Nurs*. 2001;101:26–31.

55. Campbell ML. Managing terminal dyspnea: caring for the patient who refuses intubation or ventilation. *Dimens Crit Care Nurs*. 1996;15:4–12; quiz 13.

56. Navigante AH, Cerchietti LC, Castro MA, et al. Midazolam as adjunct therapy to morphine in the alleviation of severe dyspnea perception in patients with advanced cancer. *J Pain Symptom Manage*. 2006;31:38–47.

57. Prendergast JE, Luce JM. Increasing incidence of withholding and withdrawal of life support from the critically ill. *Am J Respir Crit Care Med*. 1997;155:15–20.

58. Sedillot N, Holzapfel L, Jacquet-Francillon T, Tafaro, N, Eskandanian Ali, et al. A five-step protocol for withholding and withdrawing of life support in an emergency department: an observational study. *Eur J Emerg Med*. 2008;15(3):145–149.

59. O'Mahony S, McHugh M, Zallman L, et al. Ventilator withdrawal: procedures and outcomes. Report of a collaboration between a critical care division and a palliative care service. *J Pain Symptom Manage*. 2003;26:954–961.

60. Bakker J, Jansen TC, Lima A, et al. Why opioids and sedatives may prolong life rather than hasten death after ventilator withdrawal in critically ill patients. *Am J Hospice Palliat Med*. 2008;25:152–154.

61. von Gunten C, Weissman DE. Information for patients and families about ventilator withdrawal. *J Palliat Med*. 2003;6:775–776.

62. von Gunten C, Weissman DE. Symptom control for ventilator withdrawal in the dying patient. *J Palliat Med*. 2003;6:774–775.

63. Quill T E. Initiating end-of-life discussions with seriously ill patients: addressing the "elephant in the room." *JAMA*. 2000;284(19):2502–2507.

64. Lamba S, Quest TE, Weissman DE. Initiating a hospice referral from the emergency department. *Fast Facts and Concepts*. 2011; 247. Available at: http://www.eperc.mcw.edu/EPERC/FastFactsIndex/Documents/ff_246.htm. Last accessed January 16, 2012.

65. O'Mahony S, Blank A, Simpson J, Persaud J, Huvane B, McAllen, et al. Preliminary report of a palliative care and case management project in an emergency department for chronically ill elderly patients. *J Urban Health*. 85(3):443–451.

Chapter 11

Legal and Ethical Issues of Palliative Care in the Emergency Department

Arthur R. Derse, MD, JD, FACEP

Introduction

Years ago, emergency physicians were sometimes told that end-of-life care issues were not emergency department problems. If patients presented in extremis, "err on the side of life." Patients should be resuscitated or treated for their emergent medical problem and if treatment was successful should be admitted to the hospital; the other medical services could sort out the ethical and legal issues of end-of-life. Other adages included, "When in doubt, resuscitate—and always doubt" and "No one was ever sued for erring on the side of life." These statements are no longer true. The legal and ethical issues of appropriate implementation of life-sustaining treatment have undergone change, and as palliative care has become a subspecialty of emergency medicine, the tools and techniques of palliative care now applied in the emergency department, should be applied within the current parameters of law and ethics.[1]

To provide optimal palliative care in the Emergency Department (ED), it is important for the emergency physician to have an understanding of both the law and ethics of end-of-life care. This chapter describes the broad legal and ethical consensus concerning appropriate implementation of palliative care in the emergency department, as well as issues that lack a legal and ethical consensus. It also examines some common challenges that can arise in palliative and end-of-life care in emergency medicine. The emergency physician should be advised that the law varies from jurisdiction to jurisdiction and may change. The emergency clinician should consult with local experts for specifics of the laws as they apply to palliative care in a specific jurisdiction. Nothing in this chapter should be construed as giving legal advice for a specific fact situation.

The Interrelation of Law, Ethics, and End-of-Life Care

In the United States, the question of appropriate use of technology and end-of-life care has been the focus of significant legal developments over the past half-century. Because the focus of the issue is the initiation and continuation—or the withholding and withdrawal—of life-sustaining medical treatment in the form of various technologies, and because many of these technologies are part of the bailiwick of emergency medical practice, these concepts of law and ethics in end-of-life care must now be part of emergency medical knowledge and practice. Even though many legal cases and legislative developments in end-of-life care over the years have concerned patients who are in an intensive care or long-term care setting, most of these patients have been treated at some time in the emergency department, and the principles that have been developed are equally applicable in the emergency department. Generally the law follows medical ethical principles.

Legal and ethical issues in palliative care in the emergency department include informed consent and refusal, limitation of treatment (including do-not-resuscitate orders and other physician orders limiting life-sustaining medical treatment), determination of decision-making capacity, decision-making for the incapacitated, advance directives, guardianship and surrogates, opioids in end-of-life care, physician-assisted suicide, and futility. These end-of-life issues are generally addressed through the federal and state legislation and common (case) law through the civil court system (i.e., not through criminal law).

Because of the complex interaction between law, ethics, and emergency medicine, it is important to consider a number of issues in advance of their presentation so that when a decision needs to be made quickly, a principle of end-of-life care may be applied or an algorithm of decision-making hierarchy may be referenced. Additionally, even though many hospitals have ethics committees that provide ethics case consultation, and an ethics consultation may be a helpful possibility, many emergency department end-of-life issues arise quickly and may not be able to be considered and resolved in a timely fashion through an ethics consultation.

Informed Consent

The doctrine of informed consent is a basic tenet of American law. This legal concept is based on the ethical principle of autonomy (i.e., the patient's ethical right to self-determination) and, and with few exceptions, requires the emergency physician to obtain informed consent for testing and treatment. The emergency physician must inform patients of the risks and benefits of the procedure in question, including the alternative of no treatment.[2] In most jurisdictions, the information that must be disclosed is whatever would be material to the reasonable person in evaluating whether or not to undergo the procedure.[3] In a minority of jurisdictions, it is defined as what the professional would find material to disclose to the patient.

Emergency physicians are given authority to act without the patient's informed consent only under certain exceptions. The most common exception is known as the emergency privilege (or emergency exception) to informed consent and allows the emergency physician to act when: (1) the patient lacks decision-making capacity; (2) there is no one available who is legally authorized to act for the patient; (3) there is a serious risk of bodily injury or death; (4) time is of the essence; and (5) a reasonable person would consent (see Figure 11.1). When all

- Patient lacks decision-making capacity
- No available legal surrogate
- Serious risk of bodily injury or death
- Time is critical
- A reasonable person would consent

Figure 11.1 Elements of the Emergency Exception to Informed Consent

of these apply, the emergency physician may provide emergency medical treatment without consent. Although emergency physicians are generally aware of this exception, they may not be aware of the limited circumstances in which it applies. If there is no serious risk of bodily injury or death, or if someone is available who is legally authorized to decide for the patient, the emergency exception does not apply and informed consent must be obtained.[4]

Emergency physicians may erroneously presume that patients would want life-sustaining medical treatment under any circumstances, and institute it under that presumption. However, a number of cases have established that emergency medical treatment is like other treatments that patients may accept or refuse, and even though a presumption may be made that patients generally would want emergency medical treatment, there may be evidence to the contrary that the emergency physician is obliged to identify and honor.

Because the emergency department is often where emergency medical treatments begin, it is important to inform the patient or other decision-maker about the risks or burdens of the proposed treatment. It is also important to inform the patient or decision-maker that the intervention may be withdrawn if the treatment is unwanted by the patient (or would not have been wanted by the patient) or if the treatment is no longer working (i.e., ineffective). (See Figure 11.2) Discussing these issues and possibilities at the time of initial intervention will help facilitate better conversations with the patient and family later on. Should conversations about withholding or withdrawing treatment surface subsequently in the course of treatment, the physician can refer to these earlier discussions. Such a practice allows patients and families time to absorb these important issues as the treatment course and its effectiveness, or lack thereof, unfold.

If a patient refuses a recommended emergency medical treatment, the patient must be informed of the consequences of that refusal if the patient is willing to listen to them under the legal requirement of informed refusal.[5]

1) Ability to Understand
   a) Comprehend information
   b) Appreciate consequences
2) Ability to Evaluate
   a) Compare risks and benefits
   b) Make rational and consistent choice
3) Ability to Communicate

Figure 11.2 Elements of Informed Consent

Limitation of Treatment

In the United States, a legal consensus has emerged concerning certain principles of end-of-life care. A patient with decision-making capacity has the right to refuse any intervention including life-sustaining treatments. All patients have this right to refuse, even incapacitated patients. Incapacitated patients may have their right asserted on their behalf by a legal surrogate, such as an agent of a power of attorney for health care or a guardian. States may have specific evidentiary standards for the patient's wishes, such as "clear and convincing evidence" of what the patient would have wanted. Withdrawal and withholding of life-sustaining medical treatments are neither homicide nor suicide, and physicians' orders for withholding and withdrawing treatment are valid. Courts do not need to be involved with every case in which withholding or withdrawing of life-sustaining medical treatment is considered.[6]

This consensus emerged over a number of years of court cases culminating in the *Cruzan* case, in which the U.S. Supreme Court recognized that there is a 14th Amendment due process liberty interest that protects individuals from unwanted medical treatment. This federal legal consensus governs all end-of-life care in the United States.[7] Patients may forgo resuscitation, intubation, ventilation, artificial nutrition and hydration, blood transfusions, renal dialysis, defibrillators, pacemakers and antibiotics. All these interventions may be foregone in an emergency department setting.

Withdrawal of artificial nutrition and hydration, even though resolved legally as a medical treatment that may be forgone, may be viewed differently from some religious perspectives depending upon circumstances. Typically, decisions as to whether to begin or to stop artificial nutrition and hydration would not normally be part of emergency department decision-making.

Determination of Decision-making Capacity

Given the fact that patients may refuse even life-sustaining medical treatment, it is important to determine whether a refusal of life-sustaining medical treatment is being made by a patient who has the capacity to make this decision.

Decision-making capacity is the ability to make a specific decision about medical care. It can be contrasted with competence, which is the term used by a court to determine whether or not a person may make decisions about their person, including medical decisions, or decisions about their property, including finances. Individuals are assumed to be legally competent until determined otherwise by a court of law. The court based on expert medical opinion will often make that determination. The court, after determining a person to be incompetent, will appoint a guardian (or, in some states, a conservator) to make decisions about the person, property, or both.

In contrast to competence, decision-making capacity concerns specific medical decisions and may not correspond to the legal determination of the patient's competence. For instance, a patient who may not yet have been declared by a court to be incompetent may be determined to be temporarily incapacitated (e.g., by delirium) and might later regain decision-making capacity. As well,

1. Guardian (or conservator) of Person
2. Agent of a Power of Attorney for Health Care
3. Directions from a Living Will
4. Other Surrogates (e.g. Statutory Hierarchy)

Figure 11.3 The Elements of Decision-Making Capacity

some patients declared by a court to be incompetent may be able to express the important values that they hold with respect to medical decisions, and may even be able to make certain kinds of medical decisions.

Decision-making capacity should be routinely assessed in most emergency patients, but decision-making issues are especially acute for emergency physicians when patients refuse what seems to be treatment that would be in their best interest. Because a refusal by a patient who lacks decision-making capacity may result in the patient's death, emergency physicians need to ensure that a refusal is being made by a patient with the capacity to do so.

The decision making capacity of a patient requires the ability to receive and understand information about medical care; the ability to evaluate that information and appreciate the consequences of decision-making; an ability to apply a certain amount of probabilistic reasoning regarding the consequences of various choices; and the ability to communicate one's decision to the physician. (See Figure 11.3.) A deficiency or a break in any of these abilities constitutes a patient with a lack of capacity to make medical decisions.[8]

Decision-making capacity is task-specific. Patients may have the ability to make certain kinds of medical decisions that are more straightforward, but they may not have the ability to make more complex medical decisions. When the stakes are higher for the outcomes of medical decisions, such as those concerning life-sustaining medical treatment, the determination of decision-making capacity is even more important. Decision-making capacity is not necessarily exhibited simply by agreeing with what the physician recommends or even by making an objectively correct choice, and it certainly is not exhibited by merely expressing a preference. Some patients, such as the significantly intoxicated or the obtunded, are clearly incapacitated; however, some patients in early stages of dementia have some degree of decision-making capacity.[9]

There are a number of tests of decision-making capacity, including the popular Mini Mental Status Exam (MMSE).[10] The score on the MMSE (range = 0–30) has been correlated with clinical judgment that a patient lacks decision-making capacity. Lower scores correlate with decreased cognitive function, and at a level of 19 or less there is generally agreement that patients do not have decision-making capacity. The MMSE alone, however, or even in conjunction with other tests, may not be sufficient to determine lack of decision-making capacity. There is no professionally recognized gold standard. The determination may be aided by psychiatric or neuropsychological consultation or evaluation if there is time and opportunity.[11]

When a careful determination of decision-making capacity cannot be made in the emergency department, the emergency physician may defer an evaluation until the patient is sufficiently stabilized for a more thorough examination, but this should only be done in a case in which decision-making capacity is unclear. For patients with decision-making capacity, their considered refusal of treatment, including life-sustaining medical treatment, should prevail.

Decision-making for the Incapacitated

Once a patient has been determined to lack decision-making capacity, the emergency physician may turn to others who may be legally authorized to make medical decisions on the patient's behalf. Incapacitated patients may have a guardian (or conservator) appointed for them. That guardianship may encompass the ability to make decisions about the person, including their health decisions. Parents can be considered to be the guardians of their children's best interest until their children reach the age of majority or are emancipated through marriage, military service, or ability to support themselves, or until a court determines that the minor is sufficiently mature to make medical decisions.

Whether the incapacitated patient has a guardian, the patient may have an advance directive. An advance directive is a written document completed while the patient still is able to make medical decisions and express preferences regarding medical treatment. Completed in anticipation of circumstances where the patient may be no longer able to make medical decisions, these advance directives include powers of attorney for health care and "living wills" (also known as directions to physicians). A power of attorney for health care appoints an agent with the authority to make medical decisions according to the patient's stated wishes or based upon the knowledge of the patient's wishes. A living will is a direction to physicians that typically states that if the patient becomes incapacitated and has a terminal condition (defined statutorily) or, in some states is in a persistent vegetative state, the patient wishes to forgo life-sustaining medical treatment.

For both common types of advance directives, the patient's incapacity must be determined by two physicians, or in some states, a physician and a psychologist. In some states the power of attorney for health care must specify whether or not the patient has given the agent the ability to withdraw artificial nutrition and hydration and whether the agent may make decisions to withhold life-sustaining medical treatment if the patient is pregnant.[12]

Making decisions based on the patient's expressed (or inferred) wishes is known as "substituted judgment." If the patient's wishes are unknown, the decision-maker should use the best-interest standard, which means that the decision-maker makes decisions according to what is best for the patient under the circumstances.

If the patient is incapacitated and does not have a guardian or an agent, in some states there is a legally recognized hierarchy of medical decision-makers who may act on the patient's behalf, such as the patient's spouse, parents, adult children, or siblings, in a prescribed order.[13] In other states, there may be common law recognition of a hierarchy. In even other states, however, there is no statutory or common law decision-making hierarchy as to the appropriate decision-maker for the patient. In that case, the patient should be treated

> • Best interest (what would be best for the patient)
> • Substituted Judgement (based on knowledge of patient values and preferences)

Figure 11.4 Decision-making for the Incapacitated

according to the patient's best interests as determined by the physician's medical judgment under the circumstances, weighing input from those who know the patient's values and wishes; if there is time, a temporary guardianship may be sought to find an interim decision-maker for the patient before a permanent guardian is appointed (see Figure 11.4).

Even in cases where a patient who presents to the emergency department is incapacitated and has an advance directive, that directive may not yet be activated by formal declaration of incapacity. In other cases, the patient may have an advance directive from a state other than the one in which the emergency physician is currently caring for the patient. Even though in both situations the legal requirements for an advance directive to be valid are not fulfilled, the advance directive can provide important information to the emergency physician regarding the patient's values and wishes, and the emergency physician should take those wishes into account when making emergency medical decisions.

Do-Not-Resuscitate Orders and Physician Orders on Life-sustaining Treatment

Several mechanisms have evolved to enable physicians to translate patient wishes concerning end-of-life care into physician orders. In-hospital Do-Not-Resuscitate (DNR) orders (also know as Do-Not-Attempt Resuscitation [DNAR] orders) were developed to withhold the default action of resuscitation of a patient who experiences cardiopulmonary arrest. Do-Not-Resuscitate orders were originally devised to treat reversible cardiac arrest, but were later expanded by default to treat all cardiopulmonary arrests regardless of reversibility. Orders to withhold resuscitation were recognized as a legally valid means to withhold resuscitation from patients who did not wish it or would not benefit from it.[14]

Do-Not-Resuscitate orders initially were applicable only in the hospital setting and patients who had DNR orders and were discharged from the hospital might nonetheless be resuscitated if emergency medical services (EMS) were called for patient distress. Prehospital DNR orders were developed to allow emergency medical technicians (EMTs) and paramedics to honor DNR orders that had been written by physicians caring for the patient. These prehospital DNR orders often apply only to the prehospital and emergency department setting and are evidenced through a designated form and in some cases through a signifier worn by the patient, such as a DNR bracelet. In some cases, these orders also are considered valid in the inpatient setting. Physicians who comply with the prehospital DNR order may be immune from liability for acting in good faith upon the orders of the form.[15]

An additional, more robust, form of prehospital medical orders concerning life-sustaining treatment has been developed, known as Physician Orders on Life-Sustaining Treatment (POLST), or by a similar acronym depending upon the state in which it is authorized. These are orders issued by a physician based on the wishes of the patient or a legally authorized representative to forgo many forms of life-sustaining medical treatment including chest compressions, intubation, ventilation, defibrillation, artificial nutrition and hydration, dialysis and antibiotics. These orders carry forward through the prehospital setting into the emergency department and often into the hospital as well. Enabling state statutes may give physicians immunity from liability for acting in good faith in accord with these orders. The POLST paradigm is now prevalent in many states and EMS jurisdictions. Emergency physicians who are presented evidence of these prehospital DNR orders should act in accord with them unless professional judgment determines the orders to be inapplicable under the particular circumstances.[16]

Opioids and End-of-Life Care

Pain relief is an important objective in the emergency department, especially in end-of-life care. Many emergency physicians may be wary of prescribing significant amounts of narcotics or anxiolytics for patients, deferring pain management to the patient's primary care physician. However, patients who have a terminal diagnosis and have significant pain may need aggressive palliative care in the emergency department.

Emergency physicians should adopt practices that result in both rapid pain relief and prescription of appropriate outpatient medication for an interim period before the patient is able to see the physician treating the patient's terminal condition. The principle of double-effect states that if death is an unintended but known and unavoidable risk of appropriate pain management, and if the physician's intent is pain relief, the physician should not be held responsible for intentionally causing the patient's death should it occur as a result of the treatment.[17] Emergency physicians unwarrantedly may be concerned that they are possibly hastening death by administering these medications, but instead their actions may result in inadequate pain relief for the patient and a prolongation of the dying process.

Suicide and Physician-assisted Suicide

Emergency physicians may at times be called upon to respond to patients with a terminal condition who are brought to the ED after attempting suicide. Because there is no recognized right to suicide, if a patient with a terminal condition has attempted suicide, the emergency physician should act to reverse the conditions caused by the attempt, unless doing so would only prolong an imminent dying process.

Physician-assisted suicide continues to be the focus of great controversy in the United States. Physician-assisted suicide is defined as a physician providing lethal medication for patients to take under their own volition. Both society and the profession of medicine are divided on its permissibility. The U.S. Supreme Court has not recognized a constitutional right to assistance in suicide but has allowed states to determine their own response to this issue.[18,19] A few states allow physician-assisted suicide under specific legal constraints, and the rest of the jurisdictions prohibit this practice either by explicit statute or through common law.

In those states where physician-assisted suicide is allowed, in the unlikely event that a patient who has received assistance by a physician in accord with the law is brought to the emergency department, the emergency physician should provide palliative care to the patient. In cases where the physician is uncertain about the circumstances, the emergency physician should provide appropriate treatment until the facts become clear.

Futility

The circumstances under which an emergency physician may withhold or with-draw a life-sustaining medical treatment on the basis of its ineffectiveness is a contentious ethical issue that has not been resolved in most states. Physicians are under no obligation to provide treatments that in their medical judgment are medically inappropriate or ineffective. The mere fact that a patient or a family requests a specific intervention is not sufficient to require it. Some states have statutes that support a physician's determination of medical ineffectiveness.

Emergency physicians should exercise care in making grounded medical judgments about effectiveness of emergency interventions, and should be empathetic in communication about such judgments.

Patients who have terminal illnesses will eventually reach a point where medical treatment would no longer be effective. Though issues of futility should be addressed by the patient's primary physician in a proactive manner, this may not occur and there may be circumstances in which the emergency physician must make a determination of medical ineffectiveness on an emergent basis. In such circumstances, the emergency physician must also give the family the bad news that there are no more effective life-sustaining treatments available, and then provide appropriate palliative care. The most common emergency department determination of ineffectiveness would be in the consideration of cardiopulmonary resuscitation and other resuscitative measures. The American College of Emergency Physicians (ACEP) has stated, "[P]hysicians are under no ethical obligation to render treatments that they judge have no realistic likeli-hood of medical benefit to the patient....[For] patients in cardiac arrest who have no realistic likelihood of survival...emergency physicians should consider withholding or discontinuing resuscitative efforts, in both the prehospital and hospital settings."[20]

Summary

The laws concerning end-of-life care of patients in the emergency department are generally in accord with medical-ethical principles. Patients should be told the risks and benefits of life-sustaining medical interventions, including the fact that a treatment may be discontinued if the patient (or legally authorized surrogate) finds the treatment too burdensome or the treatment is no longer effective. Patients also have the right to refuse any life-sustaining medical treatment. That refusal should be accompanied by a description of the consequences of that refusal. Patient decision-making capacity should be assessed in the emergency department, and patients facing end-of-life who are no longer decisional may have their wishes expressed on their behalf by a guardian, by an agent of a power of attorney for health care, through the directions of a "living will," or by a legally authorized surrogate. The patient should be treated according to the patient's stated wishes or, in the absence of sufficient evidence, in the patient's best interests.

Prehospital DNR orders and physician's orders on life-sustaining treatment (POLST) are mechanisms to implement patient wishes beyond the inpatient setting. The emergency physician should administer opioids and anxiolytics as appropriate in end-of-life care. Emergency physicians may encounter patients who either attempt suicide or rarely, who have been assisted in suicide, and should respond appropriately in accordance with the law of their jurisdiction. In general, the issue of futility should be addressed proactively by the patient's primary care physician. Emergency physicians are not, however, obligated to provide medically inappropriate or ineffective treatment. Any such determination should be appropriate to the emergency department setting and carefully grounded in clinical judgment.

References

1. Quest TE, Marco CA, Derse AR. Hospice and palliative medicine: new subspecialty, new opportunities. *Ann Emerg Med.* 2009;54(1):94–102.

2. *Salgo v Leland Stanford, Jr. University Board of Trustees*, 152 Cal.App.2d 560, 317 P.2d 170 (1957).

3. *Canterbury v Spence*, 464 F.2d 772 (D.C. Cir. 1972).

4. Defenses to intentional interference with person or property. In: Keeton WP, Dobbs DB, Keeton RE, Owen DG, eds. *Prosser and Keeton on Torts.* 5th ed. St. Paul, MN: West Publishing Company; 1984:117–118.

5. *Truman v Thomas*, 27 Cal.3d 285, 611 P.2d 902, 165 Cal.Rptr. 308 (1980).

6. Meisel A. The legal consensus about forgoing life-sustaining treatment: its status and prospects. *Kennedy Inst Ethics.* 1993;2:309–345.

7. *Cruzan v Director of Missouri Department of Health*, 109 S.Ct 3240 (1990).

8. Junkerman C, Derse A, Schiedermayer D. Competence and decision-making capacity. In: *Practical Ethics for Students, Interns, and Residents: A Short Reference Manual.* 3rd ed. Frederick, MD: University Publishing Group; 2008:20–23.

9. President's Commission for the Study of Ethical Problems in Medicine and Biomedical and Behavioral Research. Decision-Making Capacity and Voluntariness. In: *Making Health Care Decisions.* Vol.1. Washington, DC: U.S. Government Printing Office; 1982:55–68.

10. Folstein MF, Folstein SE, McHugh PR. 'Mini-mental state.' A practical method for grading the cognitive state of patients for the clinician. *J Psychiatri Res.* 1975;12(3):189–198.

11. Appelbaum PS. Assessment of patients' competence to consent to treatment. *N Engl J Med.* 2007;357:1834–1840.

12. Junkerman C, Derse A, Schiedermayer D. Advance directives. In: *Practical Ethics for Students, Interns, and Residents: A Short Reference Manual.* 3rd ed. Frederick, MD: University Publishing Group; 2008:61–67.

13. Illinois Health Care Surrogate Act (Illinois Pub. Act 87–749, HB 2334, 87th Gen. Assembly, 91st Sess., 1991).

14. In re Dinnerstein, 6 Mass.App.Ct. 466, 380 N.E.2d 134 (1978).

15. Iserson KV, Rouse F. Prehospital DNR Orders. *Hastings Cent Rep* 1989;19(6):17–18.

16. Schmidt TA, Hickman SE, Tolle SW, Brooks HS. The physician orders for life-sustaining treatment (POLST) program: Oregon emergency medical technicians' practical experiences and attitudes. *J Am Geriatrics Soc.* 2004;52:1430–1434.

17. Sulmasy DP, Pellegrino ED. The rule of double effect: Clearing up the double talk. Arch Intern Med 1999;159:545–550.

18. *Washington v Glucksberg*, 521 U.S. 702, 117 S.Ct. 2258, 138 L.Ed.2d 772 (1997).

19. *Vacco v Quill*, 521 U.S. 793, 117 S.Ct . 2293, 138 L.Ed.2d 834 (1997).

20. American College of Emergency Physicians (ACEP) Non-Beneficial (Futile) Emergency Medical Interventions Policy. (Approved 1998; Reaffirmed 2002; Reaffirmed 2008). Dallas, TX: American College of Emergency Physicians Press, 2008.

Index

M